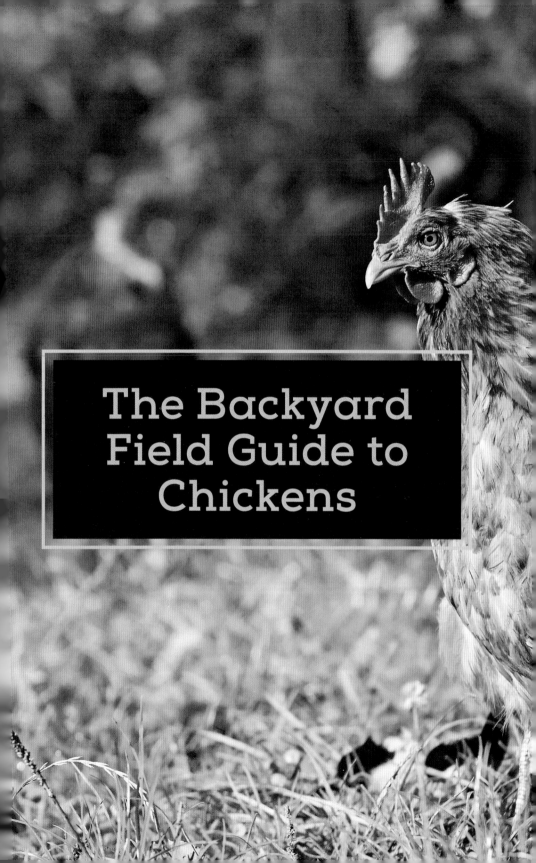

The Backyard Field Guide to Chickens

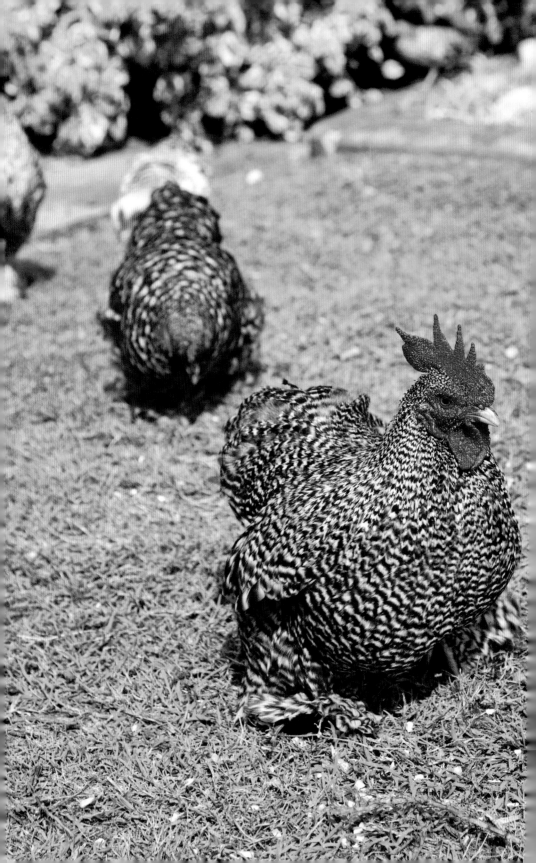

The Backyard Field Guide to Chickens

Chicken Breeds for Your Home Flock

Christine Heinrichs

Voyageur
Press

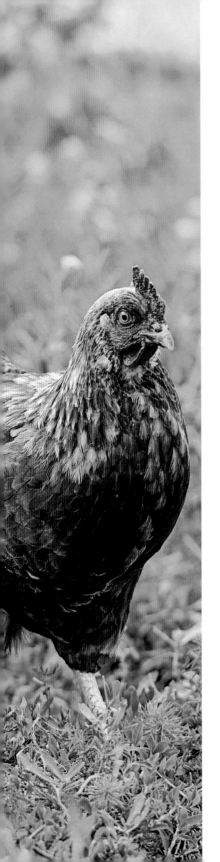

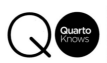

Quarto is the authority on a wide range of topics.

Quarto educates, entertains and enriches the lives of our readers—enthusiasts and lovers of hands-on living.

www.quartoknows.com

First published in 2016 by Voyageur Press, an imprint of Quarto Publishing Group USA Inc., 400 First Avenue North, Suite 400, Minneapolis, MN 55401 USA.
Telephone: (612) 344-8100 Fax: (612) 344-8692

quartoknows.com
Visit our blogs at quartoknows.com

Voyageur Press titles are also available at discounts in bulk quantity for industrial or sales-promotional use. For details contact the Special Sales Manager at Quarto Publishing Group USA Inc., 400 First Avenue North, Suite 400, Minneapolis, MN 55401 USA.

10 9 8 7 6 5 4 3 2 1

ISBN: 978-0-7603-4953-3

Library of Congress Control Number: 2016000541

Acquiring Editor: Todd R. Berger
Project Manager: Caitlin Fultz
Art Director: Brad Springer
Layout: Amy Sly

On the front cover: Imageman/Shutterstock
On the back cover, clockwise from left: bogdanhoda/Shutterstock, The Len/Shutterstock, Andrea Mangoni/Shutterstock, Kerkemeyer/Shutterstock, Annika Olsson/Shutterstock

Printed in China

Left: Chickens that eat fresh greens lay eggs with golden yolks. Green plants naturally produce yellow pigments—xanthophylls—that give yolks that bright color. *The Len/Shutterstock*

Title page: Chickens are domestic birds, descended from birds native to Asian jungles. Traditional breeds retain the ability to forage for their own food. *Lindsay Basson/Shutterstock*

Frontis: The range of red feathers is from light buff to deep, rich red colors, depending on the breed. *spiro/Shutterstock*

Contents

Introduction 6

How to Use This Backyard Field Guide 10

Chapter 1: The Road to Domesticity 12

Chapter 2: The Benefits of Keeping Chickens 24

Chapter 3: Anatomy of a Chicken 32

Chapter 4: Preparing for Backyard Chickens 42

Chapter 5: Feeding and Care 52

Chapter 6: Breed Profiles 62

Games 64

Oriental Games 70

American Breeds 84

Asiatic Breeds 110

English Breeds 124

Crested Breeds 138

Mediterranean Breeds 148

Continental Breeds 164

Other Standard and Non-Standard Breeds 184

Appendix: Glossary and Showing Information 200

Index 206

About the Author 208

Introduction

Blondie shook her white head, topped by a neatly rounded crimson comb. No floppy serrated comb for her. A compact rose comb was her crown. Her sharp hearing detected an earwig scratching in the soil. Peck, and it was history—a tasty morsel consumed.

She's a Dorking, one of my small backyard flock of ten hens. When I first started keeping chickens, back in the 1980s, I didn't think of them as a flock. They were just my chickens. Now, since chickens have attained semi-official status as the mascot of the Local Food movement, they're a flock.

Naming chickens is somewhat controversial, but when you have fewer than a dozen, it's inevitable to think of them as individuals with personalities and, eventually, names. I understand the distinctions drawn between commercial flocks of livestock and family companions. This isn't worth arguing over. Different people have different approaches to their birds.

I don't have a bone to pick with vegans who decline to use any animal products or with meat eaters who butcher their chickens and eat them. I eat chicken and prefer to buy local, but I can't imagine myself killing Blondie and eating her. Generally speaking, naming your chickens is considered the barrier to taking that final step.

Blondie came to us as an egg, shipped with eleven others from a friend in Illinois who made Dorkings a specialty. The white ones, like Blondie, are relatively new for this breed. That is, they're new since the nineteenth century, compared to Red Dorkings, which date back to the Roman Empire. Red Dorkings can be identified in Roman mosaics, accompanying Mercury, their patron god. Because the Red Dorkings have been around for so long, the Red color pattern covers a rather wide range of plumage colors.

Back in the 1800s, White Dorkings were perceived as different from other Dorking varieties, perhaps even so far as to be a different breed. In those halcyon days of Hen Fever, such points were thoughtfully argued.

Breeds have been around since humans started keeping chickens domestically, back eight thousand years ago in India and Southeast Asia. The origins of the domestic chicken remain misty, but the wild Junglefowl was too tempting a bird not to attract intense human attention. In a world without clocks, the rooster's crow started the day. As with all livestock, they

A Delaware looks the keeper right in the eye. Delawares are a solid twentieth-century composite breed making a comeback in backyard flocks. Chickens are intelligent and social. Their pecking order organizes the flock. *kay roxby/Shutterstock*

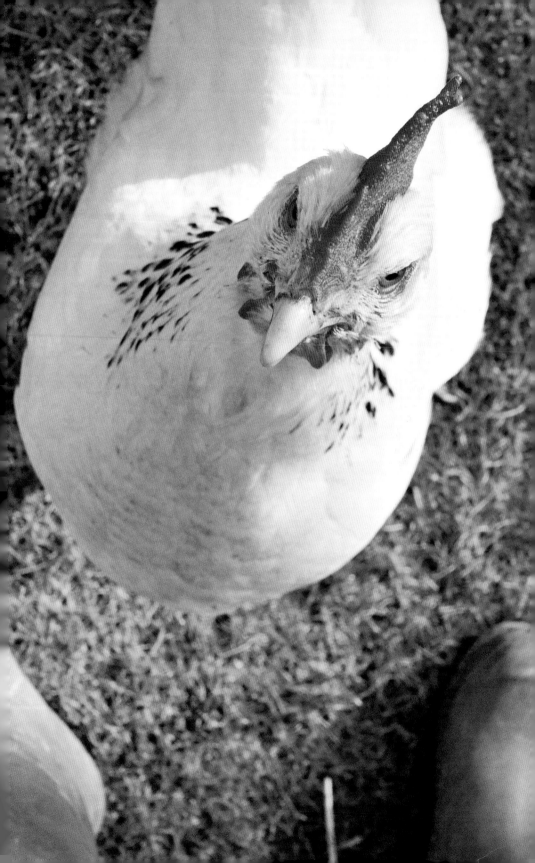

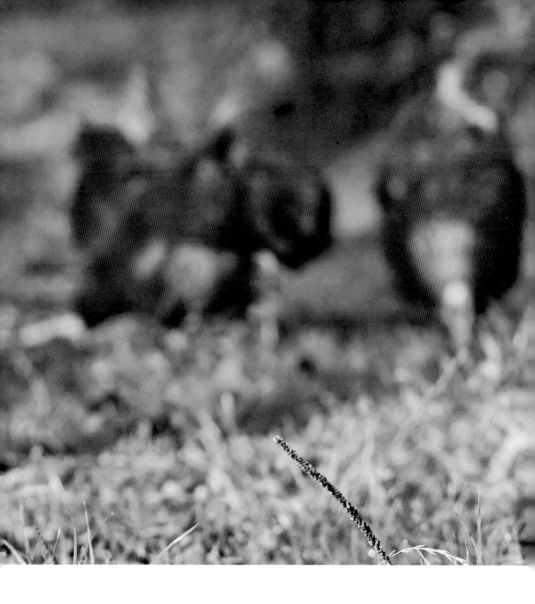

worked for a living as well as providing eggs and meat.

Their scratching and eating removed weed seeds and plant-destroying insect larvae from the soil. Their manure, scratched in as they busily work the soil, fertilized and renewed fields. Today, farmers concerned about renewing the soil and maintaining soil fertility without chemicals use chicken tractors (small, movable coops that provide the kind of soil action that mechanical tractors do,

but without the diesel exhaust) to get the same result.

Roosters' crows helped sailors find their way through the fog of Southeast Asian seas. Kept in a small cage on the bow of the boat, the sound of crowing allowed sailors to keep their boats within hearing range, and today, the Ayam Bekisar, a hybrid of wild and domestic fowl, is known for its long and musical crow. Some breeds, appropriately called Long Crowers, are known for the length of their crows, which

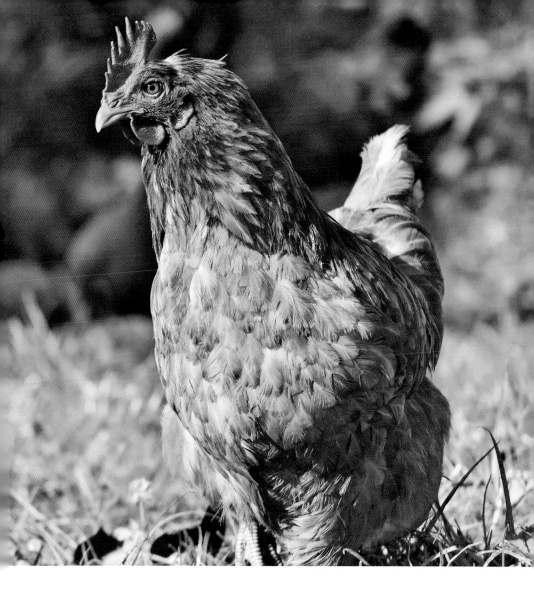

can be up to a minute long. Ah, country mornings! Suburban neighborhoods are less appreciative.

Over the centuries, poultry keepers watched the influence of selection on breeding. Poultry genetics can be confusing since breeders mate roosters and hens in every possible combination, seeking improvement in their flocks.

The many breeds that have developed in response to both the natural selection of environmental conditions and the deliberate choice of human breeders range from tiny Seramas to stately Brahmas, from Silkies to Madagascar Games. They represent the world in stunning variety.

There are no ordinary chickens. There is no perfect breed. Each is a testament to its history, geography, and beauty.

A few hens in the backyard have become popular in suburban neighborhoods as consumers look for fresh, local eggs from chickens that live good lives. *spiro/Shutterstock*

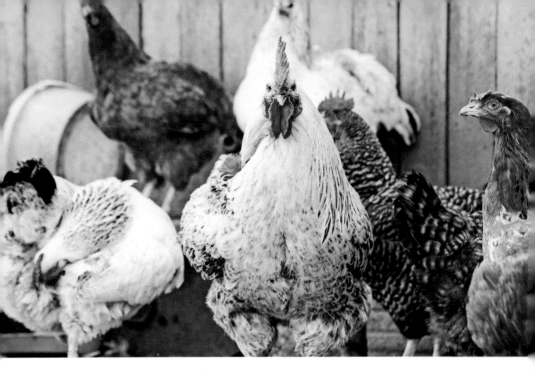

How to Use This Backyard Field Guide

Chickens aren't wild birds. You don't have to wait for them to fly overhead. They're easier to spot, perhaps even in your neighbor's backyard. You've heard them clucking. Peek over the fence and take a look.

Chances are you're looking at half a dozen brightly colored birds, scratching in the dirt. With your field guide in hand, you can identify these strange and wonderful feathered friends. That white one is perhaps a common Leghorn, but could it be a Wyandotte? An unusual sighting of a Penedesenca?

Chickens, like other domesticated critters who share their lives among humans, come in a wide variety of colors, feathers, sizes, and shapes. In the canine world, for example, you have everything from Chihuahuas to Great Danes. In the chicken world, it's bantams and large fowl, Sebrights and Malays, Modern Games and Hamburgs.

Check out local poultry shows and state and county fairs to find lots of chickens in one place. The American Poultry Association and the American Bantam Association have organized

CHICKEN WORDS AND PHRASES

A chicken with its head cut off: a lot of activity without direction. Acting hysterical or brainless.

Bad egg: an unsavory person

Good egg: a regular guy, good-natured person

Cackle: derogatory description of loud laughter

Chicken feed: insignificant amount of money

Chicken, chicken out, chicken-hearted, chicken-livered: to be cowardly

Chicken or hen scratch: unreadable and ugly handwriting

Chickens coming home to roost: to experience the consequences of one's behavior

Dumb cluck: stupid oaf

Cock-and-bull: a fantastic story that is unbelievable

Don't count your chickens until they hatch: proverb cautioning against spending assets until they are in hand

Don't put all your eggs in one basket: proverb cautioning against committing too many assets to a single investment

Egg on your face: to be caught in an embarrassing situation

Egghead: intellectual

Egg money: money raised by farm wives to supplement family income from selling eggs. Women were usually responsible for poultry flocks.

Flew the coop: left the area under suspicious circumstances

Get your hackles up: get angry or defensive

Hard-boiled: tough, street-smart

Hatch an idea: bring an idea or plan into existence

Henpecked: a husband whose wife bosses him around

Mad as a wet hen: furious

Nest egg: savings

Go to bed with the chickens, get up with the chickens: go to bed and rise early, with the sun

Mother hen: a kindly but perhaps smothering woman

Pecking order: rank, social order from high to low

Peep: tiny sound

Rule the roost: to dominate the group

Scarce as hen's teeth: so rare as to be nonexistent. Hens have no teeth.

Scratch for a living: to scrape and make do, to stretch finances

Spring chicken: youngster

Takes the cake: the winner. Plum cakes were top prizes at informal English poultry shows in the nineteenth century, often held in pubs.

Walk on eggshells: deal with a situation gingerly to avoid touching off sensitive feelings

---

chickens into detailed categories—the APA by geographic and historic type, the ABA by physical characteristics—to focus on the unique characteristics of each breed.

With your field guide in hand, you'll soon develop an eye for the subtle differences between the soft feathers of Cochins and the hard feathers of Games, the floppy comb of Anconas compared to the compact cushion comb of the Chantecler and the horn comb of the La Fleche. You'll hear the yodel of the Long Crower and the happy cluck of a hen announcing the egg she just laid. Chickens delight all the senses.

A good rooster will be a leader and protector of the flock. He is alert to possible dangers and has distinctive clucks to warn them. *ileana_bt/ Shutterstock*

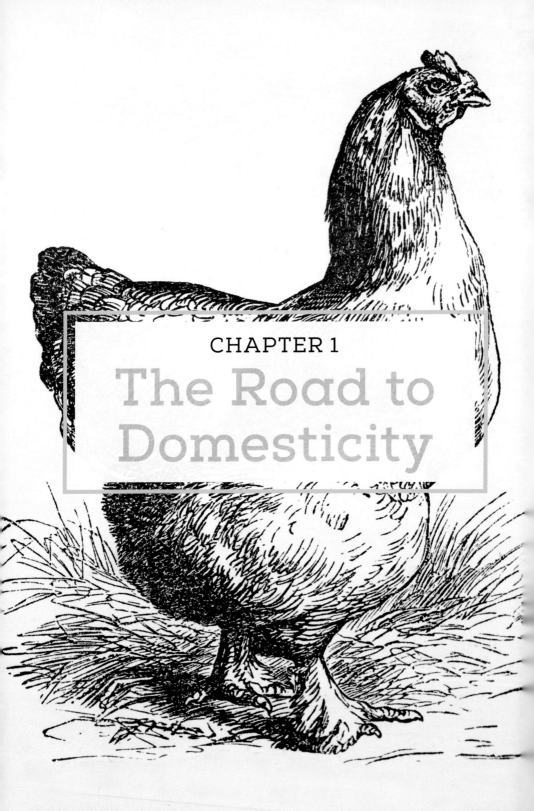

CHAPTER 1

The Road to Domesticity

As you observe chickens, you'll notice how they get around on their legs and feet. Running on those scaly legs, their three main toes scratching, their wings flapping, their beaks pecking a tasty worm—they are living descendants of ancestors of 150 million years ago. Think velociraptors. Fossil discoveries show dinosaurs with feathers, and of course, dinosaurs laid eggs. The connection gets clearer as new fossils are unearthed.

Fast-forward to fully developed birds eight thousand years ago. Junglefowl roamed the forests of India and Southeast Asia. There are four distinct kinds, but the Red Junglefowl is the main ancestor of domestic chickens. Exactly how wild, flighty Junglefowl calmed down into birds that accept human companionship still isn't clear, but domestication is a complex process, and not all animals are suited to it. Of all the thousands of species of wild animals, only about two dozen have made the adjustment. Those that have become domestic livestock had the genes to adapt. They were able to accept living close to humans, living in large groups, and reproducing in captivity. That's a crucial point, as it opens the way for humans to choose the animals that have the traits they want to keep. That selective breeding changes how chickens look and act.

As Red Junglefowl evolved into domesticated chickens, they got larger. The natural small size of wild Red Junglefowl, no larger than three pounds, suits their life. They nest on the ground but fly easily into the trees to escape predators, eat, and sleep. Their keen senses and quick response to any tiny sound that could indicate a threat keeps them safe. That wildness is a disadvantage for birds that live around people and other livestock. Now, even Red Junglefowl kept as exhibition birds are calmer. They are shown as bantams weighing less than two pounds. Large fowl chickens can be much larger, easily topping ten or twelve pounds.

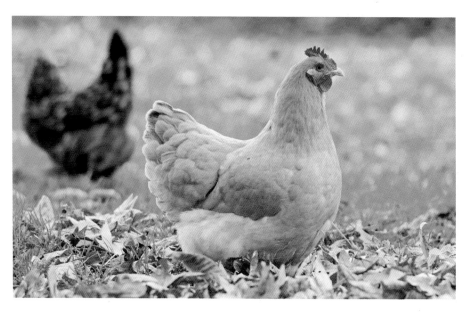

This hen's golden buff color created a sensation in the late nineteenth century when buff chickens were imported from China. It remains a popular color in many breeds. *Amy Kerkemeyer/ Shutterstock*

The bright colors of Red Junglefowl roosters are the basis of the many colors that clothe modern chickens. Junglefowl hens have the drab brown plumage that keeps them safe as they nest on the ground.

Chickens offered people good reasons to keep them around. Originally, that may have been for entertainment, such as cock fighting. Junglefowl roosters are naturally territorial toward each other, which gives them the natural aggressiveness that makes them fight. Or it may have been religious, to have the blessing of a bird that woke them in the morning, bringing the sun god and its blessings. Chickens were the guardian of Good against Evil to Zoroastrians along the Tigris River, what is now modern Armenia, in 800 BCE. Chickens are carved into altar stones excavated from Mesopotamian sites in present-day Iraq, Syria, and Turkey.

When the Persian Empire expanded across Asia and Africa around 500 BCE, chickens came with them. Greeks put chickens on coins, balancing a hen on one side and a rooster on the other. Since chickens had come from the East, the Greeks credited them with bringing the sun's light and health.

In addition to the many blessings chickens conferred on their keepers, they also laid the welcome bounty of eggs. Red Junglefowl, like all wild birds, are seasonal layers. They lay only the eggs they need to hatch and raise a family. Along the evolutionary way, chickens began laying eggs nearly every day, throughout the year.

Egyptians enjoyed chicken eggs for thousands of years, as far back as 1300 BCE. The writer Thothmes III remarked about birds that laid daily eggs, which were likely chickens. Inexpensive and easy to rear, chickens were ideal as food as well as spiritual nourishment. In Athens, Aristophanes wrote, "Every Athenian has his hen, even the poorest."

Chickens were also important for telling the future. Their behavior—if they ate or crowed—was taken as a sign of good or ill to come. Generals consulted roosters to predict whether they would win a battle. Crowing roosters pointed Athenian leader Themistocles to victory, but skeptical Cicero said, "Which is the time at which they will not crow, either night or day?"

Chicken entrails were another way to tell the future, requiring that a chicken be sacrificed, which also provided a main dish for the feast.

People found many medicinal uses for chickens. Over the centuries, specialists have described their recipes for the most effective ways to make chicken broth: using only an old rooster is a favorite. Roman naturalist philosopher Pliny, in the first century AD, recommends it, especially when made with garlic, to repel panthers and lions, among other things. Modern researchers have determined that chicken soup actually does help fight the common cold.

Chickens were probably domesticated more than once. That is, the phenomenon of domestication wasn't the brainchild of a single individual or village that then diffused by trade or other cultural contact. The attraction of wild Junglefowl could have resulted in their captivity and domestication many times in many places.

From their native home in Southeast Asia and India, chickens made their way through various cultural contacts across China and into Japan. They crossed the mountains of Central Asia to Asia Minor and into Europe. Marco Polo brought reports back to Italy from China of furry chickens with feathers like hair in the thirteenth century. The first book about chickens was written in 1600 by Ulisse Aldrovandi, an Italian scholar at the University of Bologna. He was a keen observer of the chickens he lived with

THE NITTY-GRITTY

White chickens in ancient Greece were sacred to Zeus. Fifth-century BCE philosopher Pythagoras forbade his followers to eat them.

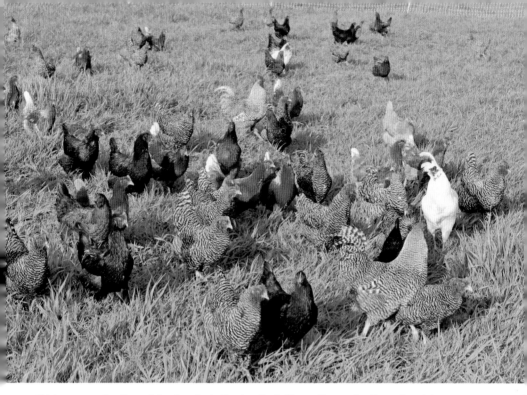

Chickens are naturally social and prefer to live in a flock. They will organize themselves into a dominance pecking order. Life in a pasture provides plenty of opportunities for even the lowest on the pecking order to enjoy life. *Weldon Schloneger/Shutterstock*

over the years, documenting many interesting chickens, such as cases when roosters raised chicks after their mother hen died. He illustrated his book with woodcuts of many unusual chickens. Chickens continued adapting to local climates and conditions in Europe and became treasured breeds.

Crossing the Pacific was a different problem. Polynesian seafarers brought chickens with them in the boats as they traveled to islands in the South Pacific. Evidence suggests that chickens lived on Easter Island and may have been brought to the mainland of South America. Archaeologists continue to explore ancient sites and identify chicken bones. Modern molecular techniques that identify DNA are adding to the birds' history.

The blue eggs of South American Araucana chickens are eye-catching. The genetic mutation that causes the blue color is also found in some breeds in China. Whether they are related remains to be determined. Whether chickens were known in South America before Europeans arrived remains a subject of discussion, but chickens spread across North and South America after the first European contact.

Selective Breeding

Many influences shaped today's domestic chickens. Breeders looked over their flocks and deliberately chose which birds to breed. That's selective breeding. Eventually, the birds they bred developed such significant and obvious distinctions that they became the Leghorns, Rhode Island Reds, and other recognized breeds raised today. In other places, birds ran free and bred on their own terms. The birds and their environment did the choosing. That's natural selection, as described by Darwin. Those birds become distinctive in their own ways, without the uniform characteristics of recognized breeds. They are called landraces and are identified with particular geographic regions, such as the Icelandic chickens.

When a flock keeper looks over his birds and decides which to keep, many qualities can go into the decision. Egg production, fast growth, and early maturation are often on the list. Resistance to local illnesses influences both kinds of selection. Birds that don't live long won't leave as many offspring as those that live long and prosper. Not all selection is for practical reasons. Some chickens are bred for looks and beautiful feathers, in color and type, that appeal to the eye and the touch. The Japanese Onigadori, for example, has been bred to grow tail feathers twenty feet long.

Chicken Breeds

What is a breed, anyway? A breed means the chickens all resemble each other enough to be readily recognized by traits that can be described. Breeds breed true—offspring resemble their parents in predictable ways. A breed has a unique appearance, productivity, and behavior. Recognized breeds are described in the American Poultry Association's Standard of Perfection and the American Bantam Association's Bantam Standard. Other countries have their own standards.

A variety is a subdivision within a breed. The chickens are similar in body type and the significant points that define them as a breed but have different feather color patterns, comb types, or another secondary characteristic.

A strain or bloodline is the result of breeding a closed flock, to which new birds have not been introduced, to the point that it develops its own identity. The APA specifies that the flock has been line bred over "a number of years." That may mean over at least five generations.

Strains are usually identified with a particular breeder, and may proudly be advertised with that name. They are chickens of a single breed and one or more varieties that are distinguished by other economic characteristics such as rate of growth, viability, size at maturity, conformation, egg production, hatchability, and feed efficiency.

Landraces are local or national breeds that develop in a geographic area that are influenced more by natural selection than intentional selective breeding by humans. They developed in response to environmental pressures and conditions and existed before people identified, named, and described them. Sumatras are an example of a landrace.

Other old breeds, considered foundation breeds, are the result of domestication and selective breeding going back centuries. They include Javas, Cochins, Langshans, Dorkings, Hamburgs, Polish, Leghorns, and Old English Games, among others. They are the breeds from which composite breeds were developed. Some of those have long histories, but some are modern, and breeders continue to cross breeds to develop new birds today. Hybrids are popular birds for backyard flocks. Show Girls, the result of crossing Naked Necks and Silkies, are a sensation at poultry shows, but not yet recognized as a formal breed.

Not all breeds are recognized. Some breeds have been dropped or are considered "inactive" due to a lack of birds being shown, such as Russian Orloffs. Others have long histories and are recognized in other countries, but not in America, such as Scots Dumpies and Dutch Brabanters.

Getting Recognized in the Standard

The American Poultry Association (APA) and the American Bantam Association (ABA) have a detailed process for recognizing a breed.

Breed clubs organize their member breeders to advocate for their breed or variety. Those advocating for the breed's recognition must submit a written account of the breed's history and the proposed standard. They must produce affidavits from at least five breeders who have raised the breed for at least five years, affirming that 50 percent or more of offspring grow up close to type.

Birds of the breed applying for recognition must be shown at APA shows at least twice each year for two years. At least two hens, two pullets, two cocks, and two cockerels must be shown.

Judges then submit their opinions of the breed and a qualifying meet is held. No fewer than fifty birds must be shown at the meet. Judges expect the birds to resemble each other closely, to establish the breed type.

HERITAGE CHICKENS

Heritage chickens must adhere to the following:

1. APA Standard breed

Heritage chickens must be from parent and grandparent stock of breeds recognized by the American Poultry Association prior to the mid-twentieth century, whose genetic line can be traced back multiple generations, and with traits that meet the APA Standard of Perfection guidelines for the breed. Heritage eggs must be laid by an APA Standard breed.

2. Naturally mating

Heritage chickens must be reproduced and genetically maintained through natural mating. Chickens marketed as *heritage* must be the result of naturally mating pairs of both grandparent and parent stock.

3. Long productive outdoor lifespan

Heritage chickens must have the genetic ability to live long, vigorous lives and thrive in the rigors of pasture-based, outdoor production systems. Breeding hens should be productive for five to seven years and roosters for three to five years.

4. Slow growth rate

Heritage chickens must have a moderate to slow rate of growth, reaching appropriate market weight for the breed in no less than fourteen weeks. This gives the chicken time to develop strong skeletal structure and healthy organs prior to building muscle mass.

Chickens marketed as *heritage* must include the variety and breed name on the label. Terms such as *heirloom, antique, old-fashioned,* and *old timey* (I would also add *historic*) imply *heritage* and are understood to be synonymous with this definition. This definition was developed by Frank Reese of Good Shepherd Poultry Ranch in Kansas in cooperation with the Livestock Conservancy.

Recent additions to the APA Standard include the Black Copper variety of Marans, the Blue Wheaten variety of Old English Game Bantam, the Splash variety of Cochin, the American Serama, the Ko Shamo, and the Nankin. In the case of the Black Copper Marans, both the color variety and the breed are new to the Standard.

New additions to the ABA include the White variety of American Serama, the Splash variety of Cochin, and the Ko Shamo.

Traditional Breeds

Traditional breeds are part of an agrarian culture that is being fragmented and lost. Traditional breeds do not flourish in industrial settings. The traits that make them special include being good foragers, good brooders, good mothers (and fathers), and alert protectors, along with longevity, disease and parasite resistance, the ability to mate naturally, and fertility.

Traditional breeds are an important part of an integrated and sustainable farm. Each breed's characteristics suit it to a climate and certain production goals. The Chantecler, developed in Canada, flourishes in a cold climate. Mediterranean breeds such as the Leghorn and the Ancona, are known for egg laying.

Choosing which birds to breed is never simple. Flocks need variability to be vigorous and avoid the pitfalls of inbreeding. On the other hand, flocks need uniformity and predictability to retain breed identity. Industrial strains seek uniformity. Traditional breeds seek genetic diversity within phenotypic (appearance) consistency.

Breed standards are mainly physical, though some are behavioral. Selective breeding is guided by breed standards. The APA specifically mentions economic value. The ABA focuses on exhibition. Conformation, plumage, comb, and color are all significant aspects of the description. Traits such as fertility, parasite and disease resistance, and longevity are less easily observed than appearance. Other heritage breeds developed as breeders selected specific qualities that suited their circumstances. Factors such

THE LIVESTOCK CONSERVANCY

The Livestock Conservancy ranks breeds according to how old and rare they are. The organization's parameters are:

- **Critical:** Fewer than 500 breeding birds in the United States, with 5 or fewer primary breeding flocks (50 birds or more), and estimated global population less than 1,000.
- **Threatened:** Fewer than 1,000 breeding birds in the United States, with 7 or fewer primary breeding flocks, and estimated global population less than 5,000.
- **Watch:** Fewer than 5,000 breeding birds in the United States, with 10 or fewer primary breeding flocks, and estimated global population less than 10,000. Also included are breeds with genetic or numerical concerns or limited geographic distribution.
- **Recovering:** Breeds that were once listed in another category and have exceeded Watch category numbers but are still in need of monitoring.
- **Study:** Breeds that are of interest but either lack definition or lack genetic or historical documentation.

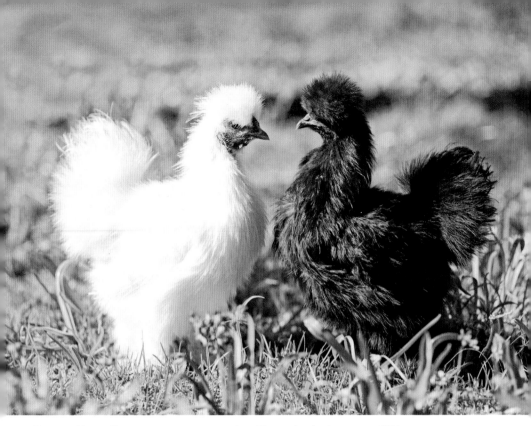

Ebony and ivory: These two roosters seem to be taking each other's measure. Silkies are among the most popular bantam chickens. See them at chicken shows in other colors as well as black and white. *Einar Muoni/Shutterstock*

as climate, kind of predators, resistance to local diseases and parasites, and the breeder's goals for the flock influenced what characteristics the breed displayed.

Choosing a Breed

All of these characteristics, along with your experience and situation, will guide which breeds are best suited to your individual circumstances. Ultimately, choose a breed you like. Bantam breeds, for example, are the introduction to chickens for a lot of people. There's a certain "wow factor" to bantams—a sweet little Silkie hen will charm even someone who thinks they don't like or are afraid of chickens. Bantam isn't a breed but an entire set of chicken breeds. They are just like full-size chickens but only one-fifth to one-quarter the size,

which means they're a good way for kids to get involved in poultry. Their small size makes them easy for small hands to manage, and most are gentler than large fowl birds. With some supervision, kids can take responsibility for care and husbandry. They are easier for children—and adults—to shampoo for a show.

Hobby breeding can save rare breeds from extinction, but to truly secure their

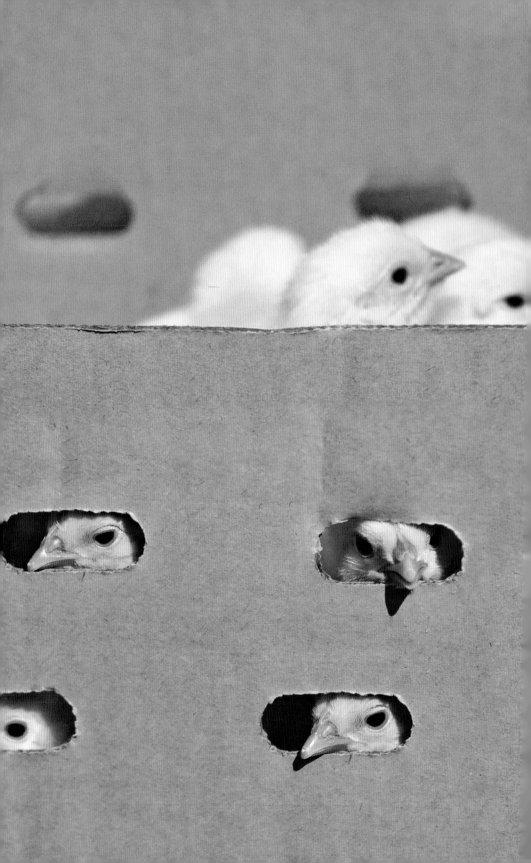

future, a market must be created for these breeds. Breeders who sell their birds and earn income will raise more of them. Having an economic purpose fulfills one of the original purposes of domestic poultry. It takes a village to save a heritage breed. Be part of history as you raise chickens! Choose traditional—this guide will help you find that special breed.

Learning More about Hatcheries and Breeds Online

The Internet is a mixed blessing, opening avenues for chicken people to connect around their beloved breeds. By their nature, many heritage breeds are kept in small numbers. Email, web pages, and social media have made communication among far-flung fanciers within reach of a keyboard.

Websites

Commercial enterprises such as hatcheries all have web pages. Many include short breed descriptions of the chickens they offer for sale. While hatchery stock may have a reputation as not meeting standard descriptions set forth by the national registries, consider your needs. If the chickens are intended for backyard pets and fresh eggs, adhering to the Standard isn't the top priority. It's better to simply get started with a breed. Even chickens that do not meet the Standard can be a good way to learn what the Standard is for each breed.

Hatcheries are doing their best to serve their customers. Providing feedback on the success of the chickens you buy from them will help them do a better job. Be a thoughtful consumer and a considerate customer.

One way to be an informed consumer is to keep records. Don't settle for obviously unsatisfactory chickens. If the Leghorns don't lay 200 eggs in a year, let the hatchery know. Heritage breeds have declined in production, but productivity can be restored with attention to production values.

Government agencies such as the USDA have web pages that offer excellent, reliable information. State extension services and university poultry departments offer information, often with local relevance for your area. Organizations such as The National FFA Organization, 4-H, the APA and the ABA have specific information about their programs.

Many breed clubs have web sites. The information on these is more reliable, because it's the product of research done by those most devoted to their breed. Enter the name of the breed into a search engine to find the breed club associated with any breed.

Nonprofit organizations such as the Livestock Conservancy have information on their programs, such as the Conservation Priority List, as well as specific breeds.

> ### THE NITTY-GRITTY
> There are about three times more chickens (about 19 billion) in the world than people (7 billion).

Chicks can be safely shipped for forty-eight hours after hatching. They need no food or water as their little bodies complete absorbing nourishment from the yolk. Large groups of twenty-five or more keep each other warm during the journey. Lucian Coman/Shutterstock

COMPARISON BETWEEN TRADITIONAL-BREED CHICKENS RAISED IN SMALL FLOCKS AND HYBRID BROILER CHICKENS RAISED IN INDUSTRIAL SHEDS

Standard-Bred Chickens	Hybrid Broiler Chickens
Anticipated life span 8 to 15 years	Minimal expected life span 5 to 12 weeks
History of thousands years	Developed in the twentieth century
Immune system fights off disease	Immune system unable to respond to pathogens
Reaches maturity in 5 to 6 months	Reaches maturity in 6 to 7 weeks
Higher cost per egg	Lower cost per egg
Lower egg production	Higher egg production
Higher cost per chick	Lower cost per chick
Many diverse breeds	Single genetically engineered phenotype
Normal walking gait	Abnormal walking gait due to short, weak legs
Can run and jump	Physically incapable of running or jumping
Can roost even as adults	Unable to reach roost
Normal, healthy weight	Morbid obesity due to genetics
Generally healthy and vigorous	Subject to disorders of heart, skin, feet, and skeleton
Mate and hatch own chicks	Incapable of natural mating or brooding
High intelligence and curiosity	Low intelligence and ability to respond to stimuli
Adapt to all types of weather	Require controlled environment to survive
Excellent foragers	Ineffective foragers
Will survive on poor feed	Require high-quality feed to survive
Smaller carbon footprint	High feed use, GHG emissions, pollution
Individuals breed their own flocks	Birds must be acquired from the corporation

News

Important news can circulate quickly on the Internet, but breaking news by definition is subject to updates. Avoid becoming Chicken Little: don't repost wild rumors. Consult fact-checking sites such as Snopes.com and FactCheck.org before passing on stories that raise eyebrows.

If you sign up for Google Alerts, a notice will automatically be sent to your email account when a particular subject is mentioned in the news.

Discussion Forums

Many Internet discussion forums or message boards on chickens welcome interested participants. Chicken questions can be posted to gather information from the assembled participants.

Social media, such as Facebook, allows like-minded chicken people to connect on group pages. Search for individual breeds to find their pages. Others focus on general interests such as backyard chickens and purebred fowl. Farms and individuals also have their own pages. If you don't find what you need, start a page.

YouTube videos range from the strange to the informative. The Livestock Conservancy has a series of videos and posts video of poultry shows. Or check out Terry Golson's HenCam and watch her hens.

Watch Out for Rotten Eggs

The Internet has its dark side. For chicken people, that includes fraudulent rare breed offers, unfilled or unsatisfactory chick and egg orders, and the echo chamber of incorrect and occasionally alarming misinformation.

Some forums are moderated, others post all entries without reading them first. Hostile and angry exchanges occasionally happen. Don't be part of one.

Be a thoughtful user and keep your "baloney detector" turned on. If it sounds too good to be true, it probably is. Check out offers for extremely rare chickens. Good breeders are always ready to provide plenty of information. Get a phone number and call and talk to them before placing an order.

FLOCK CERTIFICATION

With increased interest in heritage breed poultry, the American Poultry Association is stepping up to promote Standard breeds. Its new Flock Certification Program will certify consumer chickens, meat and eggs, and other poultry with the APA's imprimatur. Standard breeds have recognizable identity and a documented history. Reviving the certification program in the twenty-first century will help Standard breed producers justify the higher prices their products deserve.

In the past, the APA inspected flocks, but abandoned that responsibility fifty years ago. Commercial poultry farms overwhelmed smaller Standard breed flocks after World War II, and the chicken meat business turned to genetically similar, industrially developed chickens, which are unable to mate and reproduce naturally. They grow to market size in six to seven weeks, and if allowed to grow to maturity, they are hardly able even to walk. Their underdeveloped immune systems can't protect them against even ordinary diseases.

Modern hybrids with flashy names such as Freedom Ranger and Golden Nugget have been developed to take advantage of the market for chickens that are raised in better conditions. They may be raised on pasture and fed an organic diet, but their genetics often doom them to unseen internal abnormalities such as cardiac and skeletal problems.

APA-qualified judges will inspect flocks for their adherence to the APA written Standard. Judge-inspectors can offer advice to help the producer improve his flock. They can help the farmer pick out the best birds for breeding. Their knowledge, and that of the Standard breed producers they inspect, will help USDA inspectors learn how to grade Standard-bred birds.

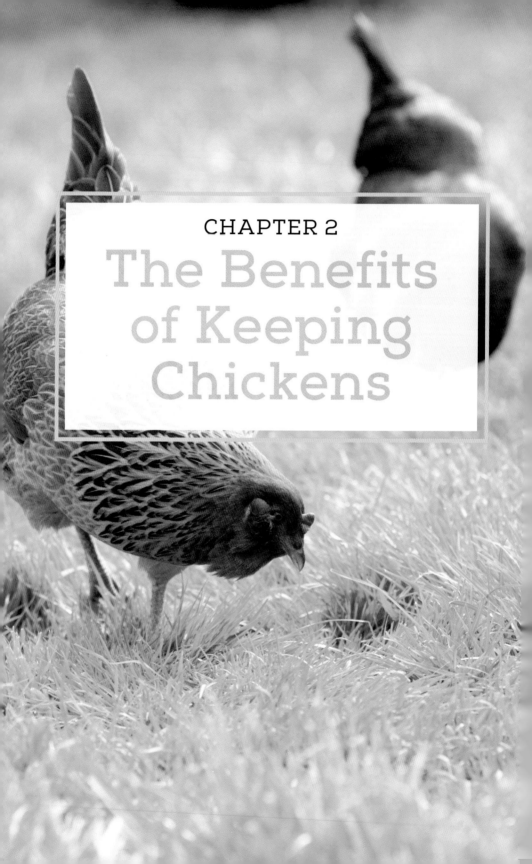

CHAPTER 2

The Benefits of Keeping Chickens

Twenty-first-century chickens in the United States don't play a part in foretelling the future. Cock fights are against the law. The chicken sold in grocery stores comes from factory farms where sheds house hundreds of thousands of chickens. But small farm owners have always kept chickens, and now backyard chickens have become the latest trend in local food, family pets, and school projects.

Backyard chicken owners often want heritage breeds. Only breeds recognized by the poultry associations are eligible for shows. Back in the day, chickens were judged for their economic value as well as their beauty. Backyard chicken owners enjoy their birds' companionship as well as those delicious eggs.

Keeping a few hens for fresh eggs is often the introduction to greater opportunities. As their interest in heritage breeds grows, owners may want to keep a small breeding flock, show their birds, or even become commercial breeders. They can all benefit from membership in poultry organizations such as the APA, the ABA, the Livestock Conservancy, and specialty breed clubs. Exhibiting chickens at poultry shows became popular in the nineteenth century, with America's first major poultry show taking place in Boston in 1849. Modern poultry shows give backyard chicken owners a chance to meet others who share their interests.

Chickens are natural recyclers. They happily eat up kitchen green waste and the occasional leftover and turn it into high-quality fertilizer. In the large quantities that come from the industrial chicken houses where thousands of birds live in their own waste, chicken manure is a pollution nightmare. In the backyard, it's part of the natural cycle of gardening. It's so valuable that people buy it in sacks from the garden shop. A small flock of hens in the backyard generates a constant supply. Chickens are also willing to scratch their own waste into the soil, an activity that the chicken tractor takes to advantage.

Disposing of waste at the landfill is expensive. Mouscron, a town in Belgium, once exceeded its limits at the local dump and was charged extra. To reduce waste, the town administration offered free chickens to residents. They offered training in successful chicken keeping—no eating the chickens—and it worked! The town's waste disposal bill was cut, and other towns followed Mouscron's example.

In the United States, the Vermont Compost Company puts hens to work on green waste and restaurant leftovers. They happily turn it into soil amendments that the company then sells to the public. The company gets eggs and meat too.

"I'm a firm believer that food will get you through times of no money better than money will get you through times of no food," said Karl Hammer of Vermont Composting Company.

Chickens have excellent vision and can spot a tasty bug or worm in the grass. *Anna Hoychuk/ Shutterstock*

Food from Your Backyard Chickens

The most obvious benefit to keeping chickens in your backyard is the fresh eggs and meat they give you, whether you keep a rooster or not. Your backyard is as local as you can get for food. You'll know what the chickens ate and how they lived.

Eggs

Every dozen eggs a backyard chicken owner gets is one less that comes from industrial caged hens, and a backyard free-range egg is more nutritious to boot. Compared to factory eggs, free-range eggs have

- ⅓ less cholesterol
- ¼ less saturated fat
- ⅔ more vitamin A
- 2 times more omega-3 fatty acids
- 3 times more vitamin E
- 7 times more beta carotene

The feeling of participation in creating local food may be reward enough, but sharing eggs at the office also has an enviable cachet. Most urban and suburban dwellers keep only hens in the yard for eggs, since roosters are often specifically prohibited. Three hens will provide a family of four with plenty of eggs.

Egg Color
Egg color is often correlated with the chicken's earlobe color. The rule of thumb is that red earlobes equal brown eggs and white earlobes equal white eggs, but there are many exceptions because egg color,

earlobe color, and feather color are not genetically linked; they are separate but distinctive in traditional breeds.

Dorkings, Redcaps, Lamonas, and Hollands have red earlobes but lay white eggs. Sumatras have gypsy-colored (dark purple) earlobes and lay white or lightly tinted eggs. Kraienkoppes are an unrecognized breed that has red earlobes and lays white eggs, and Penedesencas are an unrecognized breed with white earlobes that lays especially dark brown eggs. Araucanas and Ameraucanas have red earlobes and lay blue eggs.

Egg Breeds
All Mediterranean and Continental breeds are known for white egg production.

- Mediterranean: Leghorn, Minorca, White Faced Black Spanish, Andalusian, Ancona, Sicilian Buttercup, Catalana.
- Continental: Campine, Lakenvelder, Polish, Houdan, Crevecoeur, and La Fleche are white egg layers. Barnevelders, Welsummers, and Faverolles lay eggs in various shades of brown.
- Naked Necks are good white egg layers.
- The Australorp, an Australian-adapted English egg production breed, lays tinted eggs.
- English Redcaps are white egg producers.
- Ameraucanas are known for colorful eggs.
- Brown eggs are associated with Asiatic and American breeds.

Meat

Traditional breed chickens differ from the pale plastic-wrapped meat sold at grocery stores. Consumer attention to food quality has turned attention to these traditional breeds. The result is delicious, but some knowledge is needed to cook them well.

THE NITTY-GRITTY
The United States produces more than 50 billion eggs each year.

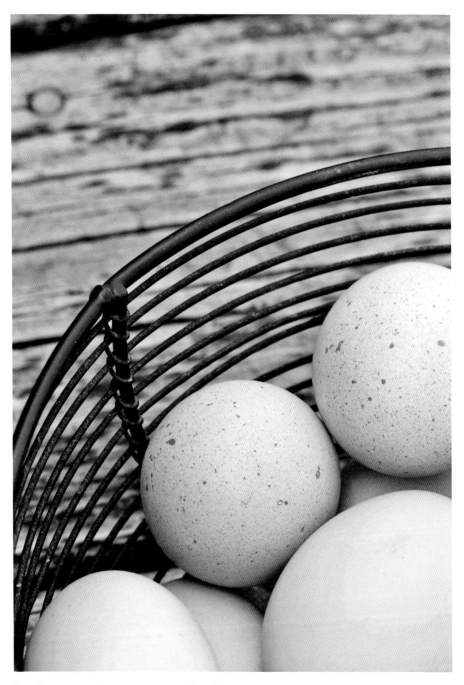

Eggs from pastured hens are more nutritious than eggs from commercial hens. They have less fat and more vitamins. Backyard chickens that enjoy better food lay better eggs. Fresh out of the hen is as fresh as an egg can be! *Stephanie Frey/Shutterstock*

"There's no such thing as tough meat," Joseph Marquette of Yellow House Farm in New Hampshire, tells students in the eco-gastronomy program at the University of New Hampshire. "Only bad cooking."

Backyard chickens that run around, live longer, and get plenty of exercise develop stronger muscles than commercial Cornish/Rock crosses. The latter live only six or seven weeks, and the only exercise they get is walking from the food dish to the waterer. Backyard chickens need to be slow-cooked over low heat to relax the meat and make it tender and tasty. High heat makes it tough.

Steve Pope, a chef working with Frank Reese's Good Shepherd Turkey Ranch in Lindsborg, Kansas, gets frequent inquiries from professional chefs for the ranch's poultry. "Chefs understand that they can use the whole bird in all their creations," he says. "They are putting their signature on their creations."

Flavor increases with maturity. A small family flock of fifty birds of a single breed could provide plenty of meat for a family for a year and sustain the flock into the following year. Chicks would hatch in March, April, and May, and be culled as they grow. For the table, chickens progress in order from broilers to fryers, roasters, and stewing fowl. A farmer would plan on keeping a dozen hens and two cockerels for the next breeding season, leaving thirty-six from that hatching season, plus older birds, for the table.

These Cochins have soft feathers that cover their legs all the way down to their feet. They get muddy in the backyard but can be shampooed to go to a show. *Annika Olsson/Shutterstock*

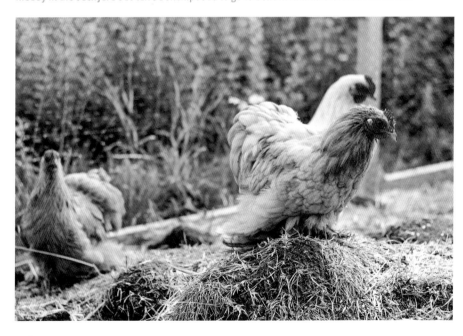

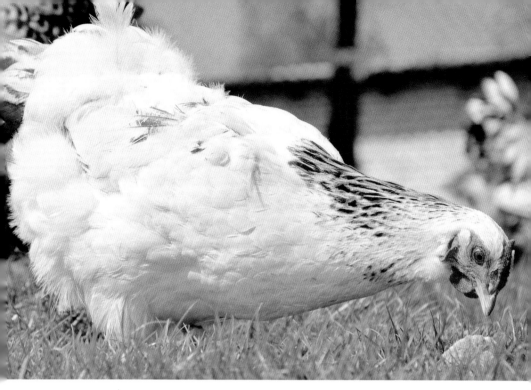

Chickens are curious but cautious. They like to explore new things, but at their own speed. This Delaware hen examines an object in the grass before taking a peck. *Tsomka/Shutterstock*

In larger breeding operations, the first birds culled are the ones with the most obvious faults that the breeder would not consider breeding. They might be culled as early as four weeks, although usually they grow to be eight to thirteen weeks old. The youngest birds, in French cuisine, are called poussin (pronounced "poosang"). Technically, this is what all industrial supermarket chicken is, killed at forty-two to sixty days old. Even flavorful traditional breeds don't have enough time to acquire much flavor in that short a time.

The meat of older traditional breed birds raised in smaller flocks is darker because the birds are stronger and better developed muscles have more oil. For the chicken, that means that their muscles work smoothly, carrying the bird through the daily routine of scratching and pecking. Because of their ancestry as upland game birds, chickens prefer to run from their predators and only fly up to their roosts. They develop dark meat in the legs and thighs and light meat in the breast.

Up until thirteen weeks of age, the birds are so young that their muscles won't flex and become tough, even when cooked under the intense heat of the broiler, hence their name. Broilers can also be fried and prepared other ways, but their significant characteristic is that they can be cooked hot and fast and still be tender.

Birds can be considered fryers from thirteen to twenty weeks, with the ideal age being around sixteen weeks. They can be cut up and pan-fried, another high-heat cooking method. They can also be spatchcocked: cut in half, the backbone and sternum removed, and the half-bird flattened then grilled. (Keep the bird away from the heat and grill at 275 to 300 degrees Fahrenheit.) Some breeds

make better fryers than others, and Chef
Pope recommends dual-purpose breeds
such as Barred Rocks and Orpingtons for
frying. They are the traditional breeds
used to prepare Southern fried chicken
for summer picnics.

Sixteen weeks is also a good time to
take a serious look at culling the breeding
flock. Quicker growing Anconas, Leghorns,
and Andalusians will show obvious flaws
by then. Slower growing Dorkings, Javas,
and Sussex need more time to develop.

In the fall, after twenty-one weeks, the
birds are roasters. Five to seven months
is the ideal age, depending on the breed.
Moist heat, provided by a cup of liquid
such as wine or broth, in a covered roasting
pan, at 325 degrees Fahrenheit, timed at
twenty-five minutes per pound, warms the
kitchen and feeds the family.

Roasters can also be dry roasted on a
spit. This method requires more attention
to baste the bird with oil to keep it moist.
Olive oil, butter, bacon, goose or duck fat,
or any other oil will do. The white meat
of the breast and the dark meat of the
thighs require different cooking times,
so a cooking thermometer is helpful for
checking doneness. Cover the breast with
aluminum foil shiny-side up to reflect
heat away and give the legs time to
finish cooking.

Older birds, the roosters culled during
the winter, or birds from previous years,
become stewing fowl. These birds have
developed full flavor and should not be
confused with industrial chickens tossed
into a pot of water and boiled. They can
become coq au vin or Grandma's chicken
soup. Slowly simmer the bird in a bath of
liquid until the meat falls off the bones.
The slow, moist heat relaxes the strong

muscles and releases flavor. The liquid
may be part of the dish, or it can be broth
used later.

Egg breeds may not have the large
carcasses of dual-purpose Buckeyes and
meat breeds such as Brahmas, but they are
delicious and should not be under-rated.

Meat Breeds

The English Cornish stands out as the
traditional meat breed. The Orpington is
second only to the Cornish.

Asiatic breeds are large and meaty, but
they are also good egg producers. Think of
Brahmas, Cochins, and Langshans for meat.

Cubalayas are renowned for their
white meat.

Dual-Purpose Breeds

American breeds are dual-purpose breeds,
large enough to be good table birds and
also laying plenty of brown eggs. Dual-
purpose breeds include Plymouth Rock,
Dominique, Wyandotte, Java, Rhode Island
Red and Rhode Island White, Buckeye,
Chantecler, Jersey Giant, New Hampshire,
and Delaware.

The old English breeds served both
purposes: Dorkings and Sussex.

Aseels are meaty and good egg layers.

Natural Compost

Chicken manure is valuable fertilizer.
Soiled litter is an excellent start to rich
compost. It needs some handling to
bring it to its best. Chickens are part of
sustainable gardening by consuming green
waste and turning it into fertilizer.

Chicken manure is high in nitrogen.
It needs to be mixed with carbon-rich
material such as sawdust, leaf litter, or
wood shavings to create the chemistry that
will turn it into compost.

Carbon-rich material includes grass
clippings, weeds, and kitchen trimmings.

The compost should be in a bin at least
one cubic yard in size that allows you to
mix the green material and soiled litter

together and wet it down. It will cook itself. The internal temperature should reach 130 to 150 degrees Fahrenheit. Let it cook there for three days. Then turn the pile, moving the material in the middle to the edges and the material at the edges to the center. Cook each cubic yard of compost at least three times this way.

Hotter is not better. If your compost reaches more than 160 degrees Fahrenheit, it will kill the beneficial organisms you want.

After you are sure it has all cooked adequately, cover it loosely and let it sit for six to eight weeks. It should be dark, crumbly, and sweet-smelling when it is ready to go on the garden.

Having two bins allows you to have one collecting soiled litter until you have at least one cubic yard to compost and one with the previous batch curing. You may want to pile the cured compost somewhere convenient to the garden.

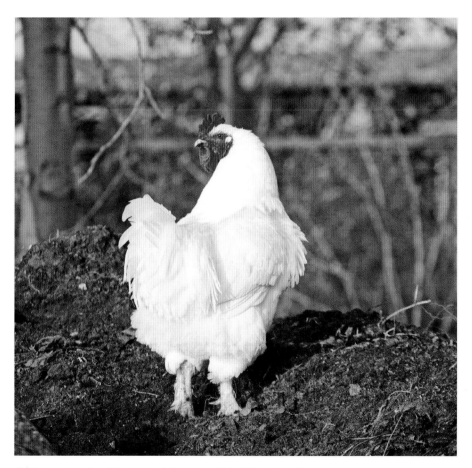

Chicken manure is a rich source of nitrogen. Mix it with compost for your garden or let the chickens work over the garden at the end of the season. They turn green waste into rich fertilizer and scratch it into the soil for you.
acceptphoto/Shutterstock

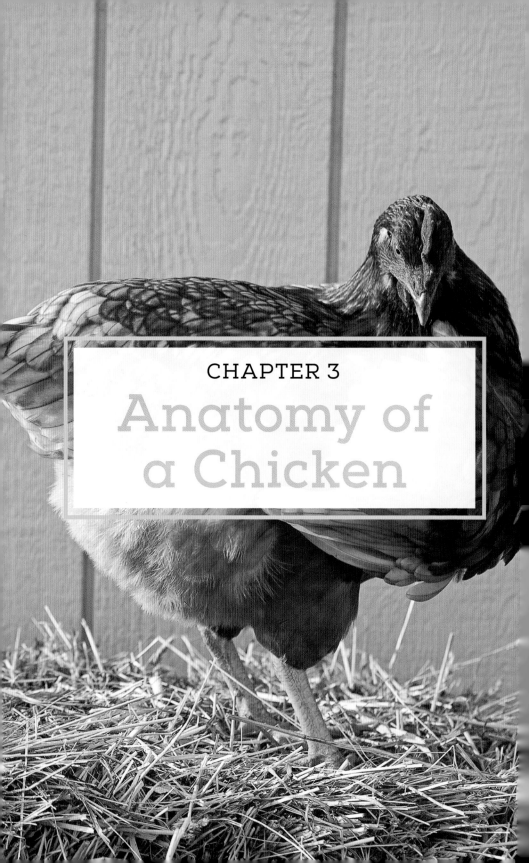

CHAPTER 3

Anatomy of a Chicken

C hickens are so varied, and the range of sizes and shapes can be dizzying, but your eye will soon pick out the identifiable differences between breeds and among individuals. Start with size, move on to feathers, then combs. You'll soon be examining feet, beak, wattles, and earlobes. All of these characteristics can be defined with technical terms: their anatomy and physiology, the finer points of feathers. This section will give you the basic facts you need to talk chickens.

Top to Toe

Look at the head. Some chickens have knobs on the tops of their heads with feathers growing out of them. Some have ear tufts growing out of the sides of their heads. Some have feathery faces, with muffs and beards.

Check the comb. Single and rose combs are most common, but combs can take elaborate shapes and sizes. Redcaps may have combs several inches long and wide. Some French breeds have *V*-shaped combs with two horns sticking up. Some combs resemble little red crowns. Small combs have the advantage in cold climates. They don't freeze the way floppy single combs do. A frozen comb will never grow back, a disqualifying flaw in a show chicken. It's also painful and debilitating for the chicken until it heals.

Wattles are the appendages that hang below the beak. Some have large wattles and some small, but whatever size they are, the two wattles should be the same. They should match the comb in color. Combs and wattles are usually red but may be purple or even black.

Chickens also have earlobes. In some breeds, they are large, in others, barely there. They are either red or white, generally corresponding to the color eggs the hen lays. Whichever color they are, they should be solid, without patches of the other color.

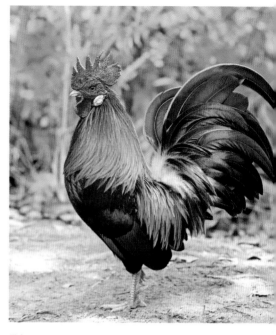

This rooster's contrasting feather colors show the different areas and types of feathers he has. His bright red single comb crowns his head, and wattles hang down under his chin. His earlobes are bright white. *PCHT/Shutterstock*

Check the beak. Chicken beaks are short and rounded, reflecting their heritage. Chickens use their beaks to peck up the seeds and insects that they eat. Beaks come in different colors, from pinkish white to black, and should be well shaped with upper and lower parts meeting so that the chicken can eat well.

Chicken legs and feet are covered in scales. The main part of the leg is the shank. Most chickens have four toes, three going forward and one going backward, but some have five, with a second toe in back. Roosters grow a spur on the back of their legs, and some hens grow them too. Spurs can be cut or broken off. The toes have a web between them, and chicken keepers sometimes use the web as a way to identify individuals by making small cut in it with a toe punch. Each toe has a toenail, which chickens use to scratch up their food.

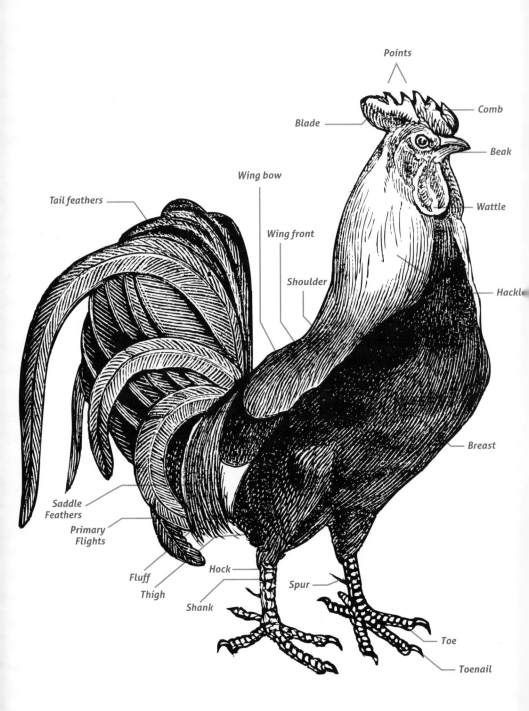

Points

Blade

Comb

Beak

Wattle

Wing bow

Hackle

Wing front

Shoulder

Tail feathers

Breast

Saddle Feathers

Primary Flights

Fluff

Hock

Spur

Thigh

Shank

Toe

Toenail

Illustration: *lynea/acceptphoto/Shutterstock*

Some chickens have clean legs, without feathers, and some have legs and feet covered with feathers. Keeping those feathered legs clean requires special care.

Feathers

Each feather grows out of a follicle in the skin. They are living tissue and should never be pulled out. The end of the feather in the skin is the quill, and the other end is the rachis. Pairs of barbs grow out of each side of the shaft. The barbs web together with tiny hooks to form the feather.

Game fowl have hard feathers. The shaft of their feathers is tough, and the feathers themselves are narrow and short. The barbs make a tight web. They don't have much fluff (the downy part near the skin).

Soft feathers are more like downy fluff, with loose webs. Cochins are known for their long, soft, lush feathers. Fanciers are so admiring that they breed them in a palette of colors and patterns. All those feathers make them look larger than they are.

Feathers may be held close to the body, as in Old English Games, or loosely, as in Cochins. Feathers are beautiful and varied, but their first purpose is to protect the chicken from the elements—they keep chickens warm in cold weather and cool in the heat and protect their skin from cuts.

Chickens care for their feathers by preening them with oil from the uropygial gland, at the base of the tail. The gland secretes an oil that keeps the feathers in good condition. They are water resistant, although not completely waterproof like duck and goose feathers are.

Feathers grow in various lengths and shapes, depending on the part of the body they cover. Each feather has fluff at the end closest to the skin, which is often a different color from the obvious outer color. The color can be important for exhibition birds.

Feathers flowing down from the head and covering the back and sides of the neck are the hackle. These feathers are special, and fishing fly-tying enthusiasts use them to make special flies. Some breeders selectively cross-breed their birds with long hackle feathers especially for the fly-tying market. Feathers from the rooster's cape and tail and hen feathers can also be used for tying different kinds of flies. The feathers on the front of the neck may be a different color from the hackle feathers. Hens and roosters of the same breed usually have different hackle feathers.

The cape feathers are the short ones that bridge the hackle and the feathers behind it on the shoulders. It looks like the chicken is wearing a cape.

The cape leads to the chicken's back, the sweep of back, the cushion, and the upper and lower saddle feathers. Behind that is the main tail. Different chicken breeds carry their tails at different angles. Some are very upright, but most are carried at 35 to 50 degrees from the horizontal.

Size, length, and color of tail feathers are the rooster's glory. Hens have tails, too, but smaller than their showy mates'. Main tail feathers are long and straight. The long flowing feathers in roosters' tails are the sickle feathers, which are also divided into main sickles and lesser sickles. Tail covert feathers cover the base of the main tail feathers in roosters. They make up most of the tail in hens. Rooster tail coverts are curved and pointed, but hens have oval tail coverts.

Below the tail is the fluff or stern and the rear body feathers. The lower thigh feathers cover the top of the legs and

THE NITTY-GRITTY

Chickens get new feathers once a year. The old ones drop out, usually at the end of summer, and new ones grow in to replace them.

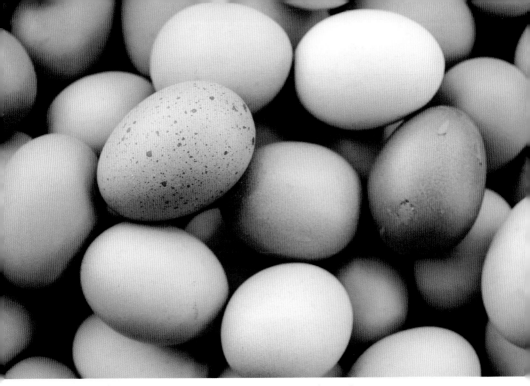

Egg color is a breed characteristic. Each hen lays the color of eggs that is in her genes. White eggs have always been popular, but brown eggs have a stylish cachet. Shell color doesn't affect the egg's nutrition, which varies according to the hen's diet. *Kentaro Foto/Shutterstock*

down to the hock plumage. The hock is the joint between the lower thigh and the shank of the leg. The feathers between the legs cover the abdomen.

Chickens' wings are divided into seven sections. The shoulder is where the wing connects to the chicken's body. The small section below that, the first part of the wing, is the wing front. Next is the wing bow, then the wing bar (covert). The secondary feathers mostly cover the primary feathers and the primary covert feathers when the wing is folded. Judges unfold the wing to examine all the feathers at shows. Incorrect feathers reduce the

points a show bird can earn, or may even disqualify it from the show, if it's a serious feather malformation, such as split wing or a twisted feather.

Although feathers help birds fly, most chickens can't fly, at least not much. Their bodies are too big for their relatively small wings to get them off the ground, though small bantams are often good flyers.

What's Going on Inside?

Chickens are different from mammals such as dogs and cats. They are omnivores, meaning that they eat a wide variety of foods, and given the opportunity, chickens love to eat worms, bugs, even mice, and lizards. Recent advertising that features all vegetarian-fed chicken raises questions

THE NITTY-GRITTY

Only one ovary functions in hens, usually the left ovary.

about how those birds get the nutrition they need.

Chickens peck up food with their beak. Although they have no teeth and don't chew the food, they have saliva, and the food is moistened in the mouth. It then slides down the esophagus into the crop. The crop is a special organ chickens and some other animals have for the next step in digestion. The crop is a muscular pouch at the end of the esophagus where food awaits digestion. After a chicken eats, you can see and feel the crop bulge with food.

The crop releases food gradually to the proventriculus, which is also called the glandular stomach, or the true stomach. This is the organ that secretes stomach acids and digestive enzymes which create chemical changes to release the nutrients in the food. The food and enzyme mixture moves into the gizzard, where the grit awaits it. The gizzard is the muscular stomach or the ventriculus, and it contracts to let the sharp-edged grit grind up the food. Grinding the food increases the surface area for the enzymes and acids to perform their chemical changes. The grit in the gizzard does for chickens what teeth do for other animals. They need a regular supply of grit in their diet to allow them to digest their food. If they are on pasture, they will pick up grit from the ground. If they don't have free access, they need a dish of grit available.

Those enzymes continue working on the ground-up mixture as it moves down into the small intestine. Enough chemical changes have been worked on the food that the nutrients are released here. The small intestine can absorb them and put them to use keeping the chicken healthy. Other enzymes enter from the pancreas. Bile is produced in the liver and stored in the gallbladder. It's added to the mix to digest fats.

The useful nutrients are absorbed as the rest passes into the large intestine. Water is absorbed here, along with any remaining nutrients not yet absorbed. Undigested food ferments in the caeca, two tubes for that purpose. The remaining material, now waste as far as the chicken's digestion is concerned, is a combination of urine and feces. Chickens excrete it together through a single opening, the cloaca or vent.

Making Eggs

The miracle of chickens is that they lay eggs regardless of whether a rooster is there to fertilize the eggs. It takes about twenty-six hours for a hen to cycle through making an egg. She won't lay at the same time every day, and won't lay an egg every day. Hen chicks hatch with the full amount of immature eggs that have the potential to develop and be laid in their entire lives.

Chickens do not lay eggs all year. All hens take some time off, usually in fall when they are molting, and in winter when the days are short. Hens respond to the length of light in a day. They need to have about sixteen hours of light, but if that much light isn't naturally available from the sun, an electric light turned on in the coop can extend the length of light in the day and prompt hens to start laying again.

Although mammals also produce young from eggs, giving birth to live offspring is very different from laying an egg and hatching a chick from it, though there are parallels between the two processes.

The eggshell functions for a chick as the womb does for a baby. It provides a protected, warm, moist place for the embryo to develop. The egg white, albumen, is a thick fluid that surrounds

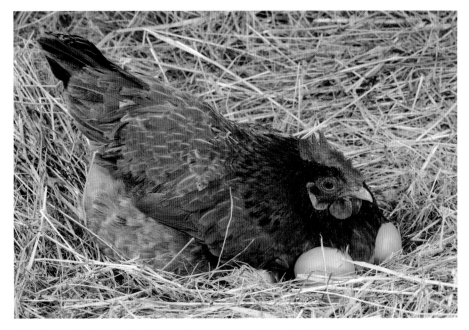

A hen is broody when she is willing to sit on eggs around the clock for twenty-one days, until they hatch. She may turn them as many as fifty times a day, to keep the embryo from sticking to the inside of the shell. *thieury/Shutterstock*

the developing embryo. It protects the embryo by absorbing shocks, much as the amniotic fluid in the amniotic sac does for a baby. The yolk is the chick's source of nourishment while it develops. In mammals, the embryo is connected to the mother by an umbilical cord. The yolk serves a similar function and carries the mother hen's antibodies.

Chicks are precocial, which means they are born ready to feed themselves. But they are not yet completely independent and need their mother to look after them and show them where to find food and water.

THE NITTY-GRITTY

A hen lays about 200 to 250 eggs a year. It takes about twenty-six hours to develop an egg to lay. The number of eggs can vary a lot by breed and individual.

Making Fertile Eggs

A rooster is a necessary part of the process for raising a brood of chicks, but both hens and rooster need to be around six months old before fertilization is possible. Hens start laying eggs when they are about four or five months old. Those first eggs, called pullet eggs, may be very small, or misshapen. They aren't fertile, even if a rooster is around. Hens can lay fertile eggs after they've had a bit of experience laying, around six months old. Roosters also need to be about six months old before they are reliably fertile and can fertilize eggs.

The rooster will mate with the hens regularly; the hen crouches down and the rooster jumps on her back, and the whole event is over in a few seconds. An overly enthusiastic rooster, or one who has too few hens to focus his attentions on, may injure the hens in his flock. He can be removed from the flock every other day to limit the time available and give the hens a chance to recover. Another option is to use hen aprons, designed to protect the hen's back. Or you can get him more hens. Adding a rooster to the flock can result in fertile eggs by the second day, but it's wise to wait four days before collecting eggs to hatch. Give him time to get around to every hen.

Hens have a "sperm nest" inside the oviduct that can hold sperm and continue fertilizing eggs up to a few weeks after the rooster is gone. So if a new rooster is introduced, it's not a certainty that he is the father of fertile eggs until about three weeks after he joins the flock.

Backyards often aren't allowed to have roosters, so fertile eggs can also be purchased from a breeder or a hatchery.

Hatching Eggs

Not every hen is willing to be broody and hatch eggs. Broodiness means your hen wants to set on eggs for the next twenty-one days, until they hatch. She wants to be a mother! She will take over one of your nest boxes and tuck in for the duration.

Broody Breeds

Because hens stop laying eggs when they are brooding, breeders have selected hens that don't get broody. Broodiness is a behavioral trait that doesn't appear in the show ring, so unless breeders want it, they may select against it. In general, show strains retain their broodiness and commercial strains do not. Bantams are more likely to be broody than large fowl.

It's a traditional trait that allows flocks to replenish themselves, so heritage breeds should be good broody hens. Heritage breeds that brood well include Ameraucana, Aseel, Barnevelder, Brahma, Buckeye, Chantecler, Cochin, Cornish, Cubalaya, Delaware, Dominique, Dorking, Dutch, Faverolle, Holland, Japanese,

Java, Jersey Giant, Kraienkoppe, Marans, Nankins, New Hampshire, Old English Games, Orloff, Orpington, Polish, Plymouth Rock, Rhode Island Red, Silkies, Sussex, Welsummer, and Wyandotte.

All games are usually good brooders. Madagascar Games, also called Malgache, are reported to be willing to adopt chicks from other broods and of different ages. Males also sometimes brood chicks.

Although hens of all these breeds are likely to be good brooders and good mothers, they vary by individuals as well. Hens can hatch any kind of eggs. You can collect eggs from other hens or even put eggs of other species under her. A good broody hen will set on them until they hatch.

The Hatching Process

A hen settles herself down, fluffing out her feathers so that she can cover the maximum number of eggs. All broody hens think big when it comes to being a mother. She'll stay there all day and all night. If you approach her, she lets out a chirping yodel of alarm. She'll peck your hand if you reach under her.

A broody hen typically gets up once a day to get a drink of water, eat, and poop. Then she's back on the nest, whether there are any eggs in it or not. Eventually, if she doesn't have any eggs to hatch, she'll get up and resume her usual place in the flock.

I like to get some fertile eggs and let my broody hens be mothers. It's a natural behavior, and the hen clearly enjoys it. One observer described broodiness as "a state of continual bliss." Writer Eva Le Gallienne described her impression of what's going on with hens in her 1949 novel, *Flossie and Bossie*. She imagines one practicing arpeggios.

Many chicken owners don't want broody hens, because they stop laying while they are brooding. Obviously, they can't be laying more eggs while they are incubating a clutch. Broodiness cuts down on egg production. So broodiness has been bred out of many breeds, which are then called non-sitters. Heritage breed flock owners usually value it. It's an instinctive behavior that allows hens to keep the flock going.

Hens, like other birds, look for some number of eggs that signals a clutch ready to be hatched. Usually, it's eight to twelve eggs. That's the reason multiple hens often take turns laying in a single nest. They are looking for that magic number.

One of the marvelous things about hatching eggs is that although an individual hen will lay one egg a day, she will keep on laying until she gets a clutch before beginning to incubate them, and then all the eggs will hatch together. This seemed like a miracle to me until I understood how they arrange it. Although some embryo development starts as soon as the hen lays a fertile egg, it won't continue until

conditions are right, with the temperature and humidity high enough to begin incubation. When the hen is off the nest, the egg is too cool for the embryo inside to begin developing. The eggs patiently wait for her to settle on them and warm them up to about 100 degrees.

Natural incubation is the traditional way to keep a backyard flock going. You will need one or more hens who are willing to set the twenty-one days required to hatch chicken eggs and a place for them to do it. Hens signal their intention to be broody by setting on the nest and refusing to move. Some hens move on and off the nest for a few days before getting serious. When a hen goes broody, she may peck at other hens who try to enter the nest to lay their eggs. When she stays on the nest for at least twenty-four hours, she's serious about it.

The hen should have a separate nest location where she can be undisturbed and undistracted by her sister hens. Keep the house clean and quiet, dark but not entirely without light, so she can see what she's doing. The eggs will cool off slightly when she gets up, which is a normal part of their cycle. The hen naturally regulates temperature and humidity; some hens pluck feathers off their breasts, to get that warmth closer to the eggs. She turns the eggs often to prevent the embryo from sticking to the inside of the shell. Hens can also be remarkably resourceful in making their own place to hatch a brood. More than one small flock keeper can tell a story about the hen they thought must have been lost reappearing with chicks surrounding her.

All this is much easier for the hen to do than for humans to replicate with an electric incubator and egg turner, but artificial incubation has been around for thousands of years. Small electric incubators are available that will hatch a dozen or so eggs, suitable for a backyard flock. Artificial incubators rely on thermometers and humidity meters.

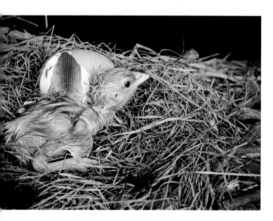

This chick has just finished the exhausting process of breaking out of its shell, but she'll soon be up and around. Chicks are ready to eat and run around soon after they hatch. *Anneka/Shutterstock*

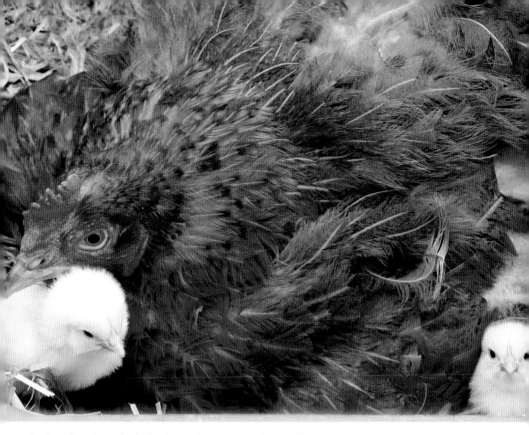

Heritage breeds retain the instinct to brood eggs and raise chicks. Hens fluff out their feathers to make plenty of room to keep chicks warm. Chicks come and go as they please. Martin Kucera/Shutterstock

Some have automatic egg turners while others rely on human hands to turn the eggs. Developing embryos exhale carbon dioxide, so the incubator must have fresh air circulation. The demands of artificial incubation may give you new respect for chickens. Once the eggs have hatched, the chicks will need special care unless a hen is willing to adopt them.

Chicks hatch by pecking a circle around the pointed end of the egg. It takes anywhere from one hour to several hours for them to get out. They peep before they hatch. For the first month of life, chicks require special living conditions provided by a brooder. In the case of naturally hatched eggs, that's the mother hen. Otherwise, a brooder can be purchased or homemade. The chicks need to be warm. They need to learn to eat and drink.

Hatching eggs is truly a miracle of nature. The mother hen will proudly show off her chicks to the rest of the flock, and the chicken keeper shares her pride and joy.

THE NITTY-GRITTY

A broody hen will turn the eggs under her about fifty times a day.

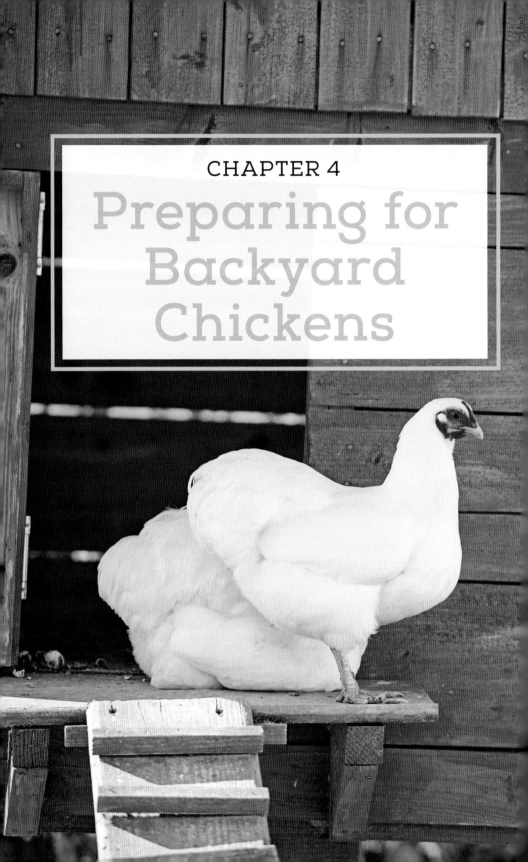

CHAPTER 4

Preparing for Backyard Chickens

Chickens are domestic livestock, so they depend on their keepers for their well-being. Their needs are simple, but unless they get the care they need, they are at risk.

As in deciding to keep any live animal such as a dog or cat, consider the future as well as the present. Taking responsibility for chickens means committing to them for their natural lives. Plan ahead to avoid unpleasant situations as chickens mature and grow old. Think through the issues presented here before making that impulse decision because the chicks are so cute.

You need to prepare for your chickens before they arrive. The rest of this chapter will outline what you should expect, including how to prepare a safe coop, how to feed your chickens, and how to keep them healthy and treat illnesses.

Starting with chicks lets them grow up more like pets. They'll enjoy being handled and come when they hear the feed dish. Some will grow up to be roosters. Roosters are seldom tolerated in backyards, so you will need to find them a new home—and that may be the frying pan. After all, these are domestic livestock developed for eggs and meat.

Young hens, called pullets, start to lay eggs at around five to six months old. The delight of finding that first little pullet egg is one of the rewards of keeping backyard chickens. They'll lay as many as six eggs a week for a couple of years. Hens slow down as they get older but keep on laying for years. Standard breed chickens have more consistent laying histories than hybrid chickens. Laying varies, but the best indicator is their breed history. Hybrids lay well for the first two years and then decline rapidly. Breeders can give you details on the chickens you buy.

Backyard chickens won't pay the bills or even compensate you for your feed and housing costs. But neither does the cat. Chickens give you delicious eggs that are more nutritious than the ones you buy at the grocery store as they enjoy a good life in the backyard. But don't expect backyard chickens to contribute financially to your family.

Hens can live to be ten years old but won't be laying many eggs by that time. Most backyard owners who keep a few chickens they have named aren't willing to butcher them and eat them, and that's usually prohibited by local ordinances anyway. Consider whether to keep chickens that are beyond their productive laying years.

Many backyard chicken keepers find that the advantages of having chickens to work over the garden at the end of the season is reward enough.

Chickens will need adequate housing and feed. Build the coop before you bring home the chicks.
The Len/Shutterstock

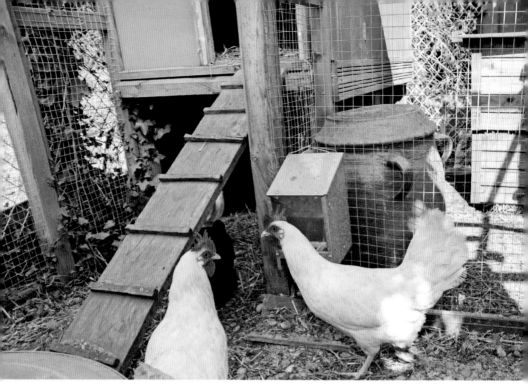

Chickens need a secure coop like this one to protect them from predators. It needs to be secure on all sides, including the ground, against animals digging under the chicken wire, and above, to protect from hawks and owls. *sylv1rob1/Shutterstock*

Chickens Are (Usually) Legal

Chickens are always are welcome in the country, but when it comes to urban areas, local regulations can vary. They are usually allowed within urban boundaries, but each governmental unit is different, so check with your local authorities. They will be able to tell you what regulations apply.

Typical urban limitations are on number of chickens, roosters (which usually aren't allowed), and how far the coop must be from houses. Many communities regulate chickens based on complaints. Getting to know the neighbors can be part of the fun. Even if you expect doubts, extending a diplomatic branch in advance sets a positive tone for future discussion. It's

rare that neighbors don't find a happy accommodation. Sharing fresh eggs generally resolves any reservations.

Another important part of being a good neighbor when raising backyard chickens is managing waste appropriately. Manure is welcome in gardens, but not when it piles up. The chicken coop shouldn't smell or attract flies. If there is more manure than the garden can use, the local garden club may welcome it.

Many people know little about poultry but are delighted to learn. Once you learn about chickens, you can be a resource to schools and local agricultural groups such as 4-H and FFA. Make yourself and your birds an asset to the community. Getting to know a network of people can also help you in the event someone challenges your right to keep poultry. Seek help and advice from people in your area and further if a legal problem develops. Pursue solutions that benefit everyone.

How to Safely and Securely Hold a Chicken

Before you can complete any up-close inspection of your chickens, it's helpful to know how to safely catch and hold one without injuring the chicken. First consider its size. Bantams are small, seldom as large as two pounds, none bigger than three. They're smaller than a small cat, and much smaller than large fowl chickens, most of which weigh in at six to eight pounds (large meat breeds can be more than ten pounds and are a real armful).

Bantams can fit on your hand. Larger birds can be held on your arm. When you catch your target chicken, put your hands on both sides so she can't flap her wings. The flapping can be alarming to the person, and the chicken could hurt a wing. Face her away from you and tuck her under your arm. Slip your free hand between her legs and hold her steady.

Practice this with friendly calm chickens who don't mind. Then you'll be prepared for the ones that view you as a fox trying to grab lunch. Roosters, for example, are natural fighters, but their keepers shouldn't tolerate any aggression toward humans. It only gets worse. If you confront an aggressive rooster flapping at you or a child, back him off with a stick or garbage can lid. Do not react aggressively toward him, as tempting as it may be. You will establish yourself as his foe, and it will only be more difficult to make him calm down. Don't attack the rooster, but keep him away. Corral him into a small area or a pet carrier, preferably a dark one. He won't like it. Eventually, he will learn that's what happens when he tries to

attack you. Reward him when he comes out with treats. That should distract him from trying to attack again.

Some have had success with carrying the rooster around for a short time, ten minutes or so, each day for a couple of weeks. It may work by establishing you at the top of the pecking order. He can't be aggressive while being firmly held.

A Safe Coop

Predators are the single worst nightmare for backyard chickens. The predator-proof chicken coop has not yet been built. Chickens need the strongest, most secure housing to foil marauders. Each location has its own local predators. It's the chicken keeper's responsibility to have strategies that keep the chickens safe.

The backyard looks serene and safe. It isn't. Raccoons and opossums are everywhere. Dogs allowed to run loose can become destructive, and domestic cats can take chicks. Coyotes, foxes, weasels, minks, skunks, and rats are not uncommon in suburbia. You may not know they are there, but they will find chickens. Snakes can take eggs and chicks. Owls, hawks, and occasionally vultures attack from above. Mountain lions and bears are rare but possible predators.

All these critters will be persistent in trying to get into the chicken coop. Protection starts with a secure perimeter. The chicken yard and coop should be securely fenced. Electric fencing can be part of the solution. The coop needs to be secure on all sides. Many predators are diligent diggers, so prevent them from getting in that way by burying fencing or having a

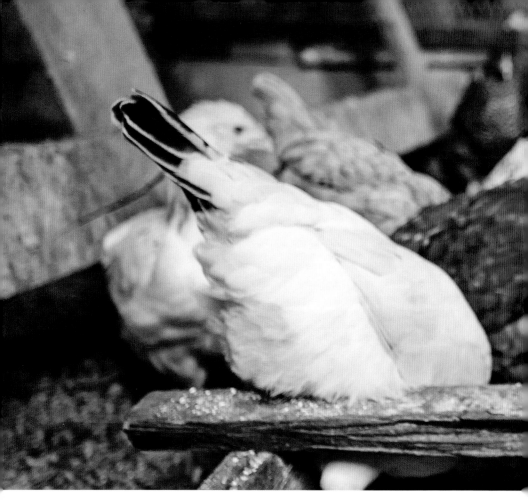

These young pullets are getting ready to starting laying eggs. Pullets are young hens less than a year old. Pullets start laying when they are about six months old. *The Len/Shutterstock*

concrete floor. Line the exterior with metal flashing around wooden structures. Birds are most vulnerable at night, so make sure the coop can be locked up.

Chicken House Designs and Features

Before you build a shelter, consider any existing structures you have, such as a play structure or space beneath a deck or staircase. Those spaces may be ready for a new life as a chicken house. A corner of the garage can become the indoor chicken house, with a run built outside. A chicken tractor is a movable coop that allows the chickens to forage safely on different parts of the yard. Use a search engine to find dozens of plans and ideas on the Internet.

In urban and suburban settings, attractive buildings and landscaping can help chickens fit in with the neighborhood. This is an example of good fences making good neighbors. Landscaping can muffle

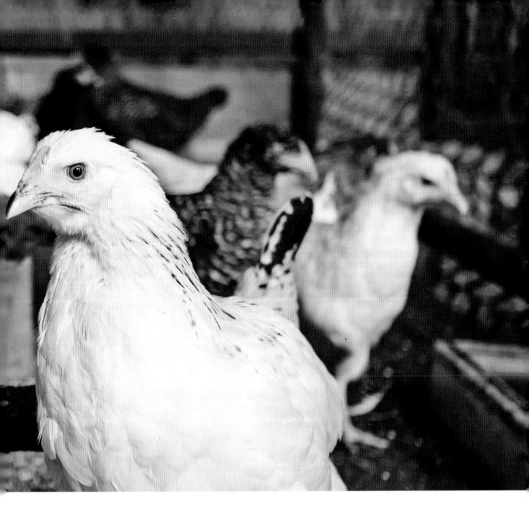

their vocalizations. Secure feed containers reduce the rodent problem.

Architecturally inclined chicken keepers design coops to complement their homes. Many cities now have annual chicken coop tours. Find out if there's one in your area and visit the coops on tour. The variety is inspiring, and everyone on the tour loves chickens.

Wood, hinges, doors, windows, and other construction materials that were previously part of other structures can be effectively given new life as parts of a chicken coop. Check with local resources for centers in your community that provide used building materials. Costs are much lower than new materials.

Ready-made or do-it-yourself chicken coop kits are available. The Eglu arrives in a box, ready to be set in your yard and welcome chickens. It is made of durable plastic with a simple and attractive design. Prices range from around $500 to $1,300.

Some assembly is required for kits. They come complete, with some options to customize for individual taste.

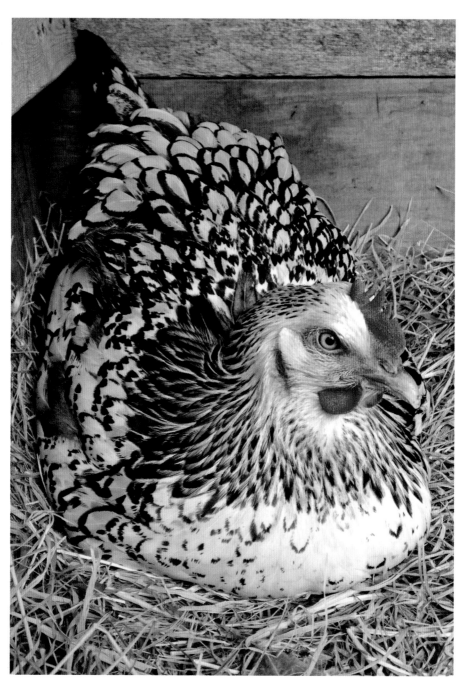

Hens prefer to lay their eggs in a nest box, and sometimes they pile on top of each other. Having a hinged back door to access the nest box from outside the coop makes it easy for the keeper to collect the eggs. *kml/Shutterstock*

Coops that are easy to clean get cleaned more often. No one wants to live near a smelly coop. Pull-out trays underneath the roosts are convenient, while deep litter systems require cleaning only once or twice a year. A deep litter system uses material such as pine shavings, leaf litter, or chopped corncobs on a dirt floor. As the chickens scratch their manure into the litter, the carbon and nitrogen mix, compost naturally, and create excellent fertilizer. The bugs that live in it add a tasty protein boost to the chickens' diet. Add litter as needed throughout the year and remove the dirt/litter/manure compost annually. Replace it with fresh dirt and litter and start over.

Chickens need shade from the heat and protection from drafts, while still having fresh air circulating. Windows allow air circulation, while protecting chickens from wind and rain. Shutters or some other way of closing windows in winter will contain the chickens' body heat and keep them warm. A line of screened vents across the

top of the north and south walls provides cross ventilation without drafts. A good coop is wind- and water-tight.

Chickens are perching birds and prefer to sleep on perches. Plan on six to ten inches of perching space per large bird. Perches can be made from 1×2-inch boards for bantams, 2×2s for large fowl, broom handles, or even natural branches. Round off sharp edges and sand rough spots.

A separate section for isolating a few chickens from the flock is an advantage. A hen with the sniffles can be treated without letting her infect the flock. A broody hen can be protected from annoyance. New hens acquired can be watched for a week or two before allowing them to join the flock, to make sure they aren't carrying any disease.

Nesting boxes provide a comfortable, private place for hens to lay their eggs. Each hen doesn't need her own—they sometimes bunk in together, and prefer to lay an egg in a nest that already has an egg in it. One nest box for every four or five hens is adequate. A wooden, glass, or plastic egg in the nest gives them the idea of where to lay. A hinged back door provides easy access for collecting eggs.

CHICKEN COOP TOURS

Backyard chicken keepers are proud of their chickens and their coops. Inviting the public along for a coop tour has become a popular way to get chicken folks together. It's fun and gives everyone a chance to exchange ideas.

Many places hold their tours in the spring, but others wait until summer or combine them with harvest events. Cities such as Atlanta, Dallas, Denver, Phoenix, Chicago, and Seattle have annual tours. Do an online search for "chicken coop tour" and your city or county to find out whether your area has one. If not, perhaps you are the one to get it started!

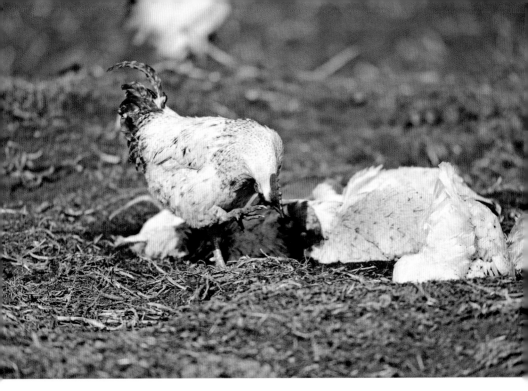

Chickens love a good dust bath. Watch them wriggle into the dirt and rub it into their feathers. When they are done, they get up and shake it all off. *Axente Vlad/ Shutterstock*

In the Chicken Yards

Chickens need a place to take dust baths. They fluff up their feathers and appear to dig their way into the ground. After they have fluffed enough dirt into their feathers, they rub their bodies against the ground. When they have done enough rubbing, they get up and shake all over.

Sand and loose dirt are the best dust-bath materials. Chickens will dust-bathe in whatever is available, but materials such as wood shavings and straw are too coarse to do a really good job. Chickens accustomed to one material may resist changing to a different one.

Dust-bathing is a natural behavior. Chicks will start bathing in their starter feed. It removes stale oil from the feathers, allowing the chicken to replace it by preening. Chickens have an oil gland at the base of the tail. Watch them touch it with the beak and spread oil on their feathers. Dust-bathing removes lice and helps control parasites.

Diatomaceous earth (DE) is a naturally occurring material composed of fossilized diatoms, a hard-shelled form of algae. It's a soft, white, chalk-like rock, pulverized for consumer use. Many chicken keepers offer it to their flock in feed, as well as in dust bath locations, to keep parasites such as lice, mites, and worms in check.

The razor-sharp edges of crystalline silica penetrate the cuticle, the outer layer of the insect's exoskeleton, causing them to dry up and die. Its sharp microscopic edges make it hazardous to breathe. Dust masks are recommended for those who come in contact with it.

Food-grade DE, the kind recommended for use with chickens, has a low percentage of crystalline silica, the most abrasive kind. (Whether it can remain in the lungs or damage the intestines has not been proven, but is a risk.)

Pecking order is enforced at the dust-bath site, but all chickens will have a chance at it. The highest-ranking chicken gets to decide when and where she will take her dust bath, then the others will take their turns.

Emergency Preparedness

Being responsible for chickens means making plans for the unexpected. An emergency plan talked through with others who are involved before disaster strikes makes coping more efficient and safer.

Any chicken keeper can be disabled or find himself in circumstances that make keeping birds impossible. Every poultry keeper needs to have a succession plan. Make a plan before events create a crisis. Chickens need someone who will take over their care if their current owner can't.

Natural disasters such as hurricanes, earthquakes, floods, and wildfires usually give some warning. Chemical spills or escaped toxic gases give no warning. Don't wait until the last minute to evacuate. Partner with neighbors or other chicken keepers to help each other in an emergency. Plan evacuation routes in advance. Have a first-aid kit that includes:

- Adhesive tape
- Antiseptic scrub
- Disposable latex gloves
- Insecticide powder (for killing biting and chewing insects on poultry, hogs, sheep, cattle, horses)
- First-aid guide

- Flashlight with extra batteries
- Gauze dressing pads
- Isopropyl (rubbing) alcohol
- Petroleum jelly
- Pocketknife
- Roll gauze
- Safety scissors (for cutting dressings)
- Scissors
- Self-stick elastic bandage, such as Vetrap
- Sterile saline solution (for rinsing wounds and removing debris from eyes)
- Syringe (without the needle, for flushing wounds)
- Tweezers
- Wound ointment/spray

In the event of a disaster, chickens will need to be contained and transported to a safe location. Have animal carriers or boxes that can accommodate them. Post the owner's name, address, and contact information on the carriers, along with the veterinarian's name and contact information and another reliable person. Pack chicken feed for the duration.

Money set aside before a disaster makes recovery easier. Keep some cash on hand and the rest in a bank.

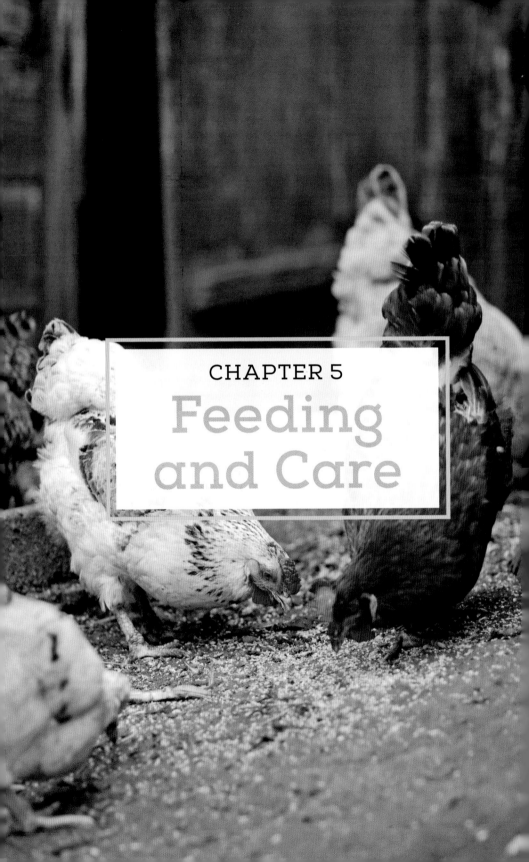

CHAPTER 5

Feeding and Care

Chickens are omnivores, meaning they eat all kinds of food, both plant and meat. They are resilient and able to thrive on a wide range of diets, but they lay more eggs and are more resistant to illness if they are getting a good, nutritious ration.

Chickens benefit from all kinds of grains, including alfalfa seed, sunflower seed, wheat and wheat germ, sesame seeds, corn, oats, rice, rye, barley, millet, flax seed, amaranth, and others. Whole grains and seeds are better than cracked since they contain oils that are necessary for good feather condition and carry important vitamins for good health. Corn, wheat, and oily sunflower seeds in particular supply protein.

Commercial feed is a good way to start with chickens; many companies and some local feed mills make their own formulations. Oils are added to commercial feed to replace those lost in processing. Manufactured feed is inevitably more processed and older than feed you make yourself, so as you gain experience as a backyard chicken keeper, you can learn more of the refinements of poultry nutrition and move on to making your own feed. Some people even sprout grains like wheat, oats, barley, and rye for their chickens. (Seeds can be soaked and sprouted on trays lined with moist paper.)

Chick starter is around 20 percent protein. Chicks are usually kept on starter for at least sixteen weeks, or until about half the flock of that age are laying eggs. Backyard chicks are often started with feed medicated with Amprolium or Bacitracin, to help them acquire immunity to coccidiosis, a protozoan parasite with microscopic eggs that live in the dirt. It is not an antibiotic and works by limiting the chick's uptake of vitamin B1, which the protozoa need to multiply. Because it doesn't kill the parasite outright, the chick develops its own lifelong immunity to coccidiosis. Medicated feed isn't necessary if coccidia aren't present.

Chicks should grow steadily. Some breeds grow more slowly than others but should be vigorous and steadily gaining weight. Chickens can get too fat, however, which can interfere with laying. Hold them in your hands and feel for a fat pad between the legs. If it's cushy, they are too fat. Gradually reduce the amount of grain or other carbohydrates in the diet.

Chickens gather round the feed dish. The pecking order is subject to change, but each chicken knows where he or she stands in relation to the others in social ranking.
Alex_Po/Shutterstock

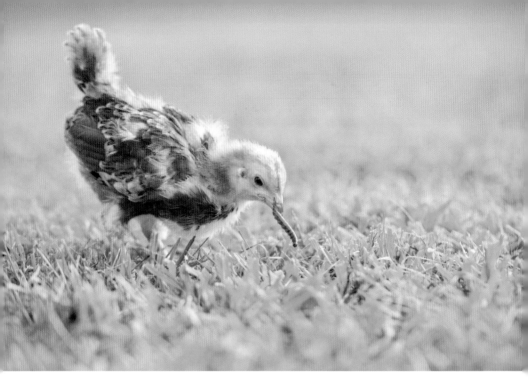

Chicks need feed that helps them grow all those feathers and gives them a good start in life. Commercial feed is nutritionally balanced, but the thrill of catching a tasty worm adds joy to a chick's life. *eurobanks/Shutterstock*

After using starter, transition your chickens to grower and then layer crumble or mash. An average laying hen will consume about one-quarter pound of feed, four ounces, per day. Obviously, larger birds will eat more than tiny bantams. Mash and crumble can be messy, spilling out of the feeder, creating unsanitary conditions and attracting rodents. Feeders with an extra lip over the feeding trough or protected by a grill reduce spilling. Wall mounted or hanging feeders in more than one location help entertain confined birds. Multiple feeders offer birds low in the pecking order ways to get enough to eat.

Fish and fish meal, worms, and insects of all kinds are tasty treats that chickens enjoy eating. Each has its own balance of nutrients, so know what your chickens need and are getting. Small flock owners have satisfied their flocks with everything from trapped yellow jackets to fly maggots and earthworms. One of my chickens was a regular companion when I weeded the garden, taking advantage of the tasty worms I dug up. Snails, a problem in some areas of California, were so plentiful that the chickens became blasé about a new shipment. My gardening neighbors used to bring my chickens pails of them to get rid of them. Feed stores also carry insects such as dried mealworms. My hens run out when they hear the plastic bag crinkle.

Greens give chickens vitamins and minerals as well as fiber. They enjoy grass and weeds of all kinds, and will happily eat up your garden if they can get into it. Any garden waste makes an interesting challenge for chickens, since they are attracted by new things in their yard. Clean grass clippings and weeds also make good greens, but make sure the lawn clippings haven't been subjected to fertilizer and herbicides.

Green kitchen cuttings are wonderful chicken food as well. Additional greens can usually be found at your local grocery store. Ask for produce trimmings; some produce managers will give them to you free or for a nominal charge. Large bags of trim will delight backyard chickens. These fresh greens and other interesting food options such as hanging corncobs or seaweed in their enclosure give them something to do. Bored hens can start bad habits, such as picking at each other's feathers or eating their own eggs.

Chicken scratch is a supplement, not a full diet. Scratch feed contains cracked grains like corn, wheat, and sorghum. Scratch is the traditional supplement to barnyard chickens that ranged to forage for greens and insects and received plenty of kitchen scraps.

Chickens love leftovers and will eagerly eat spaghetti and hamburgers. Be mindful that a lot of prepared foods include salt. Though it's a necessary nutrient, chickens can die from too much salt, and more than

0.15 percent salt in their diet will cause soft-shelled eggs.

Chickens prefer clean water and will avoid fouled water. They may stop eating if they don't have clean water to wash down their food. Waterers should be washed frequently and rinsed with bleach every week or two.

A contentious topic is the addition of antibiotics to commercial feed. Antibiotics are one of the advantages of modern medicine, but adding them to feed has been linked to producing antibiotic-resistant strains of bacteria in commercial animals. Industrial chicken operations add antibiotics to the feed to increase weight gain and feed conversion, but constant

HERBS

Raw garlic is a popular herbal preventive and remedy. Many chickens like it. Feed it to chicks so that they can acquire a taste for it.

Tobacco has a long history as a medicinal for many ills of humans and animals. In fact, the nicotine in it is a powerful poison, making tobacco an effective parasite control. Adding tobacco leaf stems to nesting material may reduce mites and lice. A nice handful of chewing tobacco serves the same purpose. It won't hurt them if they eat a bit, and may help control worms.

Pennyroyal is the smallest of the mint group, with a pleasant and noticeable aroma. It gets its scientific name, *Mentha pulegium*, from *pulex*, the Roman word for flea. Pliny records that the Romans used it against fleas. Pennyroyal makes another excellent nesting material that will keep your chickens free of lice and mites.

Any aromatic herbs make good nesting material. Peppermint, spearmint, catnip, oregano, wild bergamot, lavender, rosemary, sage, basil, thyme, and fennel may grow wild or can be cultivated in gardens. The scent in herbs comes from natural oils that may inhibit germs. Nettle, alfalfa, lamb's quarters, and dandelion are other tasty and nutritious herbs chickens enjoy. Check with a local herbalist for specific recommendations.

feeding of subclinical doses—less than is needed to cure infection—produces antibiotic-resistant strains of bacteria that can then infect humans.

Keeping Your Chickens Healthy

Just as in humans, a long list of varied diseases and disorders plagues chickens, but most of the time, illness is caused by a few familiar bugs. If your chickens do get sick, they will most likely recover, and backyard chicken keepers are usually able to manage the occasional sick chicken on their own with supportive care. Any sick chicken that does not respond within a few days, however, or causes rapid spread of illness through the flock, requires professional veterinary attention.

The best defense against disease is for the flock to be clean and well nourished. Clean, fresh water and food stop disease before it can spread. Dirty water breeds pathogens, and chickens are smart enough to avoid dirty drinking water, but then they can become dehydrated. They will also stop eating if they do not have water to drink. It's a downward spiral that makes them vulnerable to any germs lurking around the coop.

Fresh air and sunshine are the best disinfectants. Give your chickens plenty of space since crowded conditions breed problems. They should have room to roam. Crowding causes stress, which reduces their ability to resist disease or recover if they do catch something. Crowding increases the speed and reach of disease spread. Birds that have more space are less likely to catch diseases from each other.

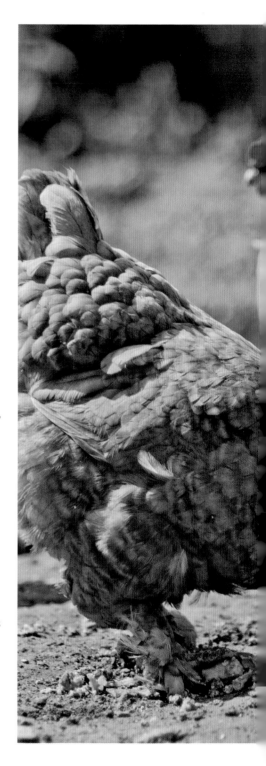

Chickens are natural foragers. They enjoy picking through kitchen trimmings and garden waste for tasty scraps. *Kemeo/Shutterstock*

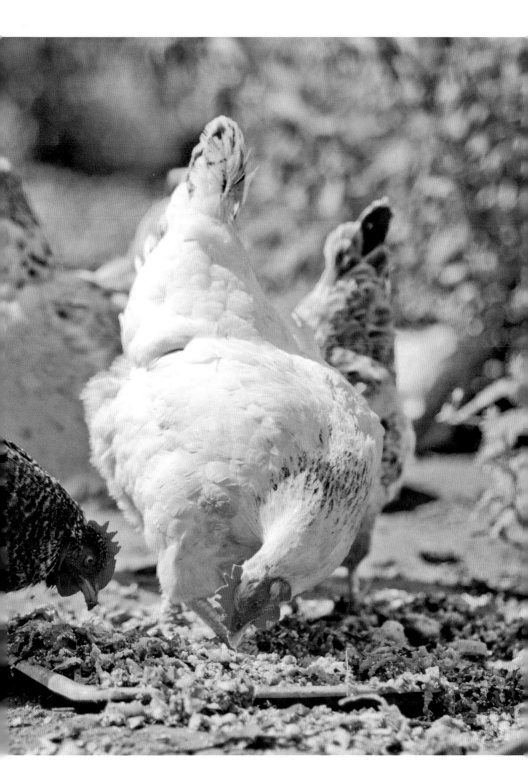

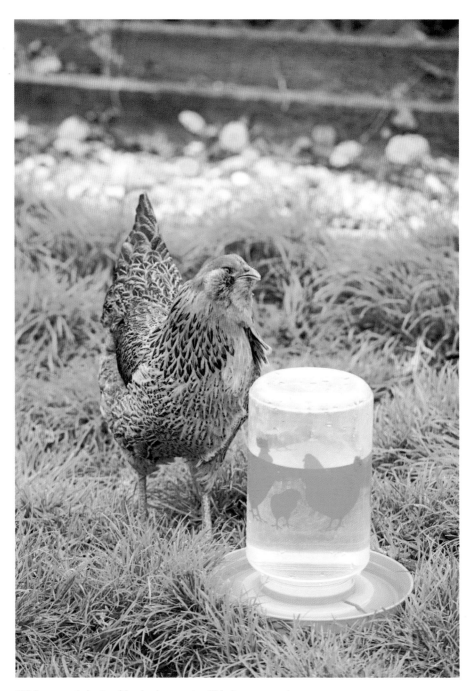

Chickens need plenty of fresh, clean water. This Ameraucana hen, noted for her muffs and beard, looks forward to refreshing herself at the waterer. *Anna Koychuk/Shutterstock*

A backyard flock should allow at least one and a half to two square feet per chicken inside the hen house and eight to ten square feet of yard outside. Bigger is better. Chickens need space to stretch their wings and interact socially with each other.

Backyard flocks can be small, three to five hens, but not fewer than that. Chickens are flock birds. They need each other to establish a social pecking order. Solitary chickens sometimes adopt the family cat or dog, just to have some social life.

Control rodents in the housing and yards, as they can carry diseases and parasites.

The poultry yard needs to drain excess water so that it won't become a breeding ground for mosquitoes, bacteria, or parasites.

When using any chemical treatment, whether an antibiotic or other medicine or an insecticide, read and follow all package directions.

Biosecurity

Backyard chickens are among the most biologically isolated critters in our world, in the sense of contacting micro-organisms that may make them sick. Be aware of which diseases have been a problem to other poultry owners in your area and take appropriate precautions. Avian influenza is the most notorious, but birds can share other diseases.

Diseases can be spread by dirt, feathers, and other items that carry infection with them, as well as by live birds. Simple biosecurity practices, however, can stop them at the front gate. Make a habit of washing your hands before and after handling birds. Backyard chicken keepers can easily keep a pair of garden shoes at the back door. Using only those shoes to visit the chickens stops most contamination right there. Inexpensive disposable

boot covers can allow neighbors to be welcome visitors without compromising flock security. A jacket that is only used for gardening and the chickens is a second line of defense. I wear old clothes when I clean the chicken coop and then toss them in the washer.

Keeping records of biosecurity measures will help you respond in the event of a disease outbreak.

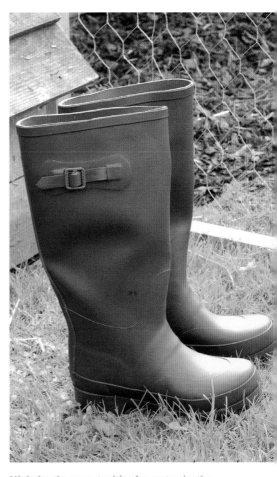

Minimize the opportunities for contamination by keeping boots you use only in the backyard. Then you won't be tracking in potential disease. Chickens are generally healthy, but disease occasionally strikes. *tezzstock/Shutterstock*

Remember also to exercise caution when introducing new chickens to your flock. Acquire birds only from sources that can verify that they are disease-free. Then quarantine new birds for ten days to two weeks in separate quarters, to assure that they are healthy.

Chickens Don't Sweat

Normal body temperature for a chicken is 105 to 107 degrees Fahrenheit. That's higher than many viruses can withstand. It may explain why chickens don't get certain livestock diseases, such as anthrax. Their jungle origins make them able to thrive even in hot times, tolerating temperatures up to 100 degrees Fahrenheit with relative humidity of 65 percent. They don't sweat, but they will pant when they are hot. They reduce body heat by breathing out warm air. They may also hold their wings away from their bodies. Make sure they have a cool shady place to escape the heat.

When Chickens Get Sick

Avian influenza (AI) takes many forms in birds, some of which are more devastating than others. Low pathogenic forms of AI circulate through the poultry community. Just as in people, healthy backyard chickens may get the sniffles, or even a more serious case, but generally they recover without incident.

Cases of a new highly pathogenic strain of avian influenza that showed up in North America in 2015 were confined almost entirely to large, crowded commercial flocks. Those conditions are quite different from the living conditions of backyard chickens. HPAI can pass rapidly through birds confined in close quarters as they are in commercial operations, transmitted by sneezing, coughing, and touching. The crowded conditions of commercial poultry operations are also ideal for the mutation of low pathogenic influenza into highly pathogenic forms.

Influenza viruses mutate constantly. The 2015 strains, H2N2 and H2N8, infected only poultry. The H5N1 strain that began affecting chickens in 2003 occasionally infected people, but none in North America. AI is unlikely to affect a flock in suburbia, but it gets a lot of public attention. Fears of bird flu should not discourage anyone from keeping backyard chickens.

The virus does not survive long outside the chicken. It isn't a danger to food. Cooking kills it, as does hand washing.

Chickens occasionally contract other diseases. Coccidiosis is a parasitic disease that can affect any kind of birds. Most chick feeds include a preventive medication. Birds develop immunity as they encounter the organism that causes it.

Chickens can get lice and mites, and once those pesky critters show up on feathers, a chemical insecticide treatment will be needed to get rid of them. Get professional advice from the local livestock extension person, an experienced breeder, or a veterinarian.

Chickens can carry salmonella bacteria without being sick themselves. Salmonella can make people sick, so don't kiss chickens, and wash your hands after handling them. Refrigerate eggs and eat them well cooked.

Despite your careful plans, predators that study the landscape may find a way in and injure a chicken. Most minor injuries and infections can be successfully treated with triple antibiotic ointment, bandages, and tape. Flexible adhesive bandaging such as Vetrap is useful and difficult for even a determined bird to remove.

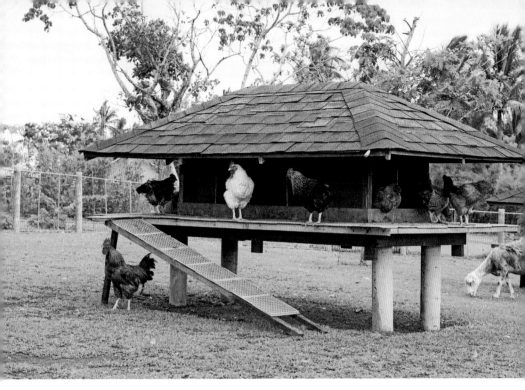

Chickens get along well with other livestock. They can reduce parasites that affect sheep and goats by eating the worms that afflict them on pasture. Large livestock can also keep predators away from chickens. *richardernestyap/Shutterstock*

Petroleum jelly is useful for treating scaly leg mites and can help prevent frozen combs.

Antibiotic use is best reserved for sick or injured chickens. Industrial chicken operations add low doses of antibiotics to regular chicken feed because chickens gain weight faster when they eat antibiotics every day. No one knows why this happens, but chickens that grow faster reach market weight sooner. This isn't a concern for backyard chickens. Feeding antibiotics every day produces antibiotic-resistant strains of bacteria. When they infect chickens or people, the usual antibiotics aren't effective. Antibiotic-resistant infections are a serious medical problem. Backyard chickens don't need to add to it.

Veterinary Advice

Having a relationship with a veterinarian who is willing and able to care for chickens before they get sick is an advantage. Chickens are a specialty that not all are prepared to treat. Other poultry owners in your area can recommend individuals. *Backyard Poultry Medicine and Surgery, A Guide for Veterinary Practitioners*, is a resource manual to support general practice vets who want to learn how to care for chickens and other poultry.

Contact veterinarians and discuss your situation with them before you have a sick chicken crisis. Local veterinary advice can help you make decisions on vaccination and other preventive measures for your flock.

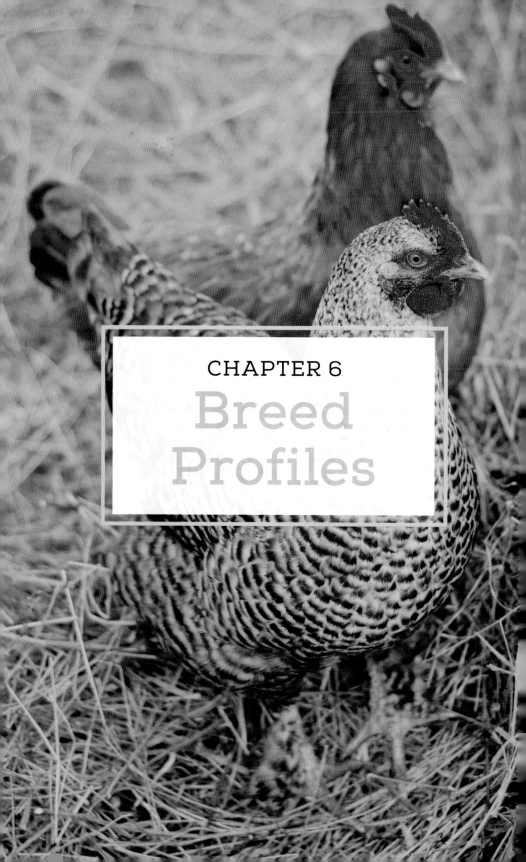

CHAPTER 6

Breed
Profiles

As you visit neighbors' yards, community gardens, and farms, notice how different the chickens are. Some are white, some black, then all colors, brown to gold, solid and spotted, some with heads one color and the body another. Roosters and hens of one flock may look very much alike, while others are entirely different colors. Some are big; some are tiny. Some have feathers all the way to the ground, some have feathers all over their faces, some have topknots, some have no feathers on their necks at all.

As your eye for the differences develops, your skill at identifying breeds grows. This section will help guide you to recognizing which breed you are watching. Each breed description includes the key differences of one breed from another.

All chickens trace their lineage back over eight thousand years to Asian Junglefowl, but because chickens are domestic livestock that have been kept for household use, their keepers have bred them for specific characteristics. Chickens have also been more independent in the past than they now are and have adapted to their living conditions through natural selection as well. Chickens traveled with explorers over the centuries, coming from India and Indonesia to China, across Asia to Turkey and the Middle East, to Africa and Europe. They came across the Pacific with Polynesian islanders to Easter Island, perhaps to South America.

The result is the panoply of chicken breeds from around the world that now live in American backyards.

The APA and the ABA are the certifying organizations governing poultry exhibitions. They write and approve the breed standards and train judges to evaluate birds brought to shows. It's a great system for describing and qualifying birds, getting every breeder onto the same page as to what is the best bird.

Not all the birds you will see have been blessed by the qualifying process. Breeds may be more popular in their home countries and never had enough following in the United States to meet the rigorous requirements for official recognition. Their breeders may simply never have organized to make the effort. Not being recognized in the standard isn't a judgment of worthiness. The world of chicken breeds is varied and active; additional breeds are always in the process of applying for recognition, and breeds that are no longer being shown may be dropped for lack of participation.

Chickens have varied plumage. The black-and-white cuckoo pattern can camouflage a bird in dappled sunlight and shade. Selective breeding over the centuries has developed colors to suit every climate and aesthetic taste. *bogdanhoda/Shutterstock*

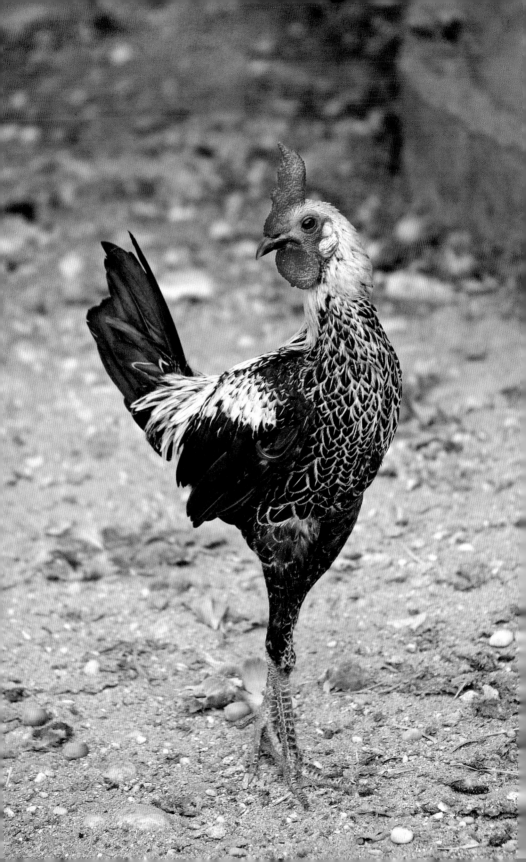

GAMES

The Games are the oldest, original breeds of domestic chickens and take their name from their history as fighting chickens. Setting animals to fight each other to death is a blood sport that lost mainstream acceptability. While there are illegal cock-fighting rings in the United States, it is now against the law in every state. It continues to have ethnic followings.

Games have been so revered through the centuries that the palette of breeds and colors is beyond limit. The Old English is the classic image of the chicken. Modern Games are lithe and graceful, modern art on two legs. American Games have taken their own path, away from their European forebears, while Oriental Games trace a more direct ancestry to India and Asia. Cornish, known for its meaty build, was originally called the Indian Game.

Games are hard-feathered birds. Their feathers are glossy and fit closely to the body, and they have fewer feathers than soft-feathered breeds. The Oriental Games may have bare spots on their bodies, especially on the neck and breast.

Games have brought with them across the centuries their distinctive dignified walk and their stately carriage. They have a haughty eye, daring a challenge to their rule of the roost. Games are ready to defend their homes and families, and that fighting instinct has its origin in protecting the vulnerable from jungle predators. Many Games retain their fighting disposition. Their inclination to fight makes it necessary to separate them, in some cases into individual pens, and even the chicks will pick fights with each other.

While Games have been selected for courage, agility, and strength, they are not inherently vicious. Selection for strength is what has produced their excellent table qualities.

Old English and Modern Games are recognized by both the APA and the ABA as separate breeds. Among bantams, Old English Games are the most popular single breed. American Game bantams are recognized by the ABA. Large fowl American Games are not APA-recognized but have passionate advocates.

Games are among the most popular breeds. Their name refers to their history as fighting chickens. Blood sports are no longer admired or even legal in the United States, but the fine birds that developed along the way earn honors at poultry shows. *Andrea Mangoni/Shutterstock*

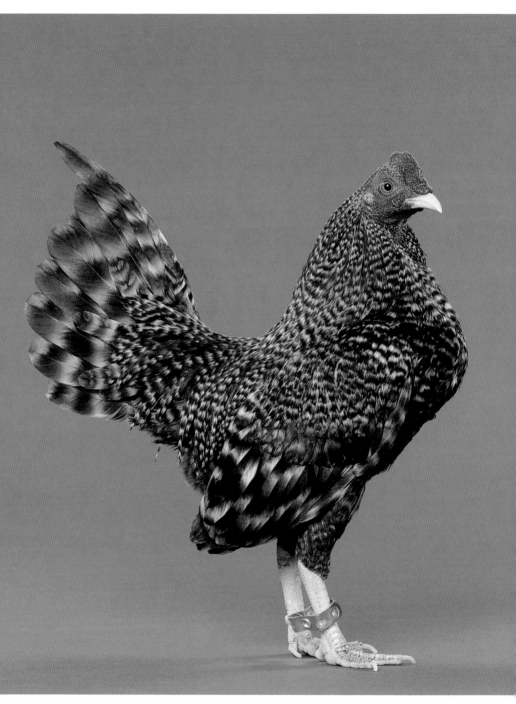

The special barred color pattern on this Old English Game Bantam rooster is called Crele. Clearly marked bars on Crele chicken feathers win in the show ring. *Derek Sasaki/www.mypetchicken.com*

OLD ENGLISH GAME

The Old English Game is the iconic chicken of nursery rhymes and chicken decor. The flowing feathers of the traditional Black-Breasted Red Color pattern glisten orange, red, green, and iridescent black that catches the sun, shimmering with flashes of red, purple, blue, and green.

Old English Games are docile and easily managed. The males fight only other male chickens, and the hens get along well together, fighting only to defend their nest or brood of chicks.

Old English Games are the chickens of the English countryside as well as early America. They are the homestead fowl, good layers, and tasty meat birds who could find their own food and take care of themselves. In the United States, Old English Games were the utility small farm chickens into the early twentieth century.

With such rich ancestry, all colors are possible, and breeders along the way have raised them all. As a result, more than 170 color and pattern variations have been documented. Black-Breasted Red is the traditional color, but solid colors such as white and black and other color patterns such as Golden Duckwing and Red Pyle brighten the chicken yard and the show ring. Fanciers maintain a wide variety of colors that aren't recognized by any official standard.

With all those varied birds in their background, other feather variations show up. They may have muffs—feathers around the front of the throat—or tassels—feathers growing from the back of the head. The tassel is often called a toppie (TOE-pee), and it isn't a true crest but a small cluster of feathers at the base of the comb. Both the muffs and tassels hark back to Old English Games of centuries past.

Hen- or henny-feathered roosters, sometimes called "lark-feathered," look like their hens. They have the reputation of being fast and cunning fighters. The British Poultry Club recognizes these variations and many American breeders cherish them.

Old English Games are required to be dubbed for showing, meaning the comb and wattles are surgically removed. This gives them the traditional look of fighting fowl. The original purpose of the practice was to prevent the other rooster from getting a grip and gaining an advantage. Unless they are going to be exhibited, Old English Games do not need to be dubbed.

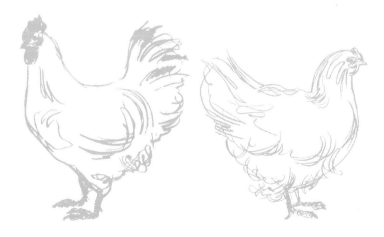

MODERN GAME

Modern Games are different from all other chickens. They stand tall, slender, and graceful, whether large fowl, which weigh up to six pounds, or the tiny bantams, at no more than twenty-two ounces. Their shape and the way they carry their body is called "station."

Modern Games have been around since the 1800s, and eight color varieties were included in the APA's first Standard of Excellence in 1974. Only one more has been added since, in 1981. So "modern" is relative comparing their ancestry to the ancient heritage of other game chickens. Breeders who loved their Games when they were fighting cocks turned their attention from the pit to the show ring after cock fighting was outlawed. They bred Malays with Old English Games and refined the result to produce the Modern Game.

Their feathers, like other Games, are hard and short. Exhibitors polish them with a silk cloth before the judge sees them at the show.

Like Old English Games, the roosters must be dubbed, their comb, wattles, and earlobes cut off, for showing. This is usually done at about eight months old. Removing the comb and other headgear gives the birds a more streamlined appearance.

They are adequate layers and some are good broody hens, but those who love them keep them for showing. They were developed to be admired. They are curious and friendly and make good pets.

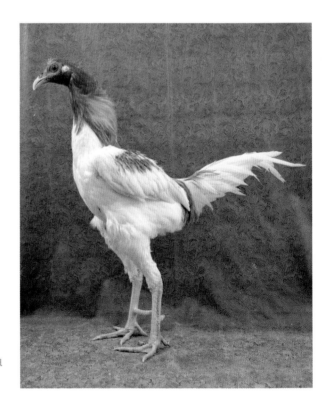

Modern Games are not ordinary barnyard chickens, although they are as hardy as their backyard cousins. They are usually bred for the show ring rather than their practical usefulness. *Courtesy of the Livestock Conservancy*

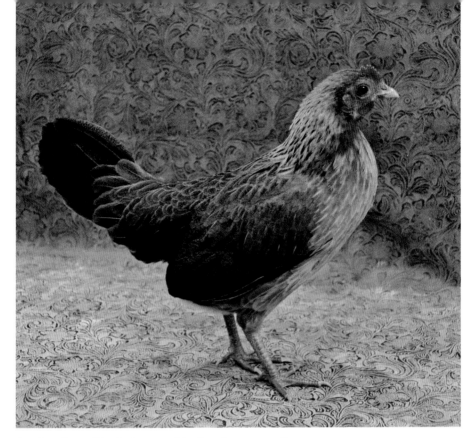

American Games like this hen are said to have been among the chickens kept by George Washington, Abraham Lincoln, and Andrew Jackson. *Courtesy of the Livestock Conservancy*

AMERICAN GAME

American Game chickens have more plumage, larger tails, longer wings, and a different body shape from Old English Games. The bantams have a longer back than the short-backed Old English Games and carry their tails higher. Their feathers are longer and more lush, with curled sickle feathers. American Game Roosters keep their long tails as they age. Most have bluish slate legs, some black or pinkish slate.

American Games stepped away from their European and Asian background over the years. They were bred as fighting birds and their passionate advocates admire their vigor and strong disposition. Bantams are raised for the show ring and are recognized by the ABA, but large fowl are not yet recognized by the APA. The American Game Fowl Society has its own standard.

Beginners are warned off starting out with American Game large fowl. Their gladiatorial attitude toward life, and anyone they deem to be an intruder, requires experienced handling. Bantams, on the other hand, can be a good choice because they are so hardy.

Both large and bantams are strong and resilient. Breeder Anthony Saville describes them as "tough, proud, bold, and fearless chickens to be admired for their resilience."

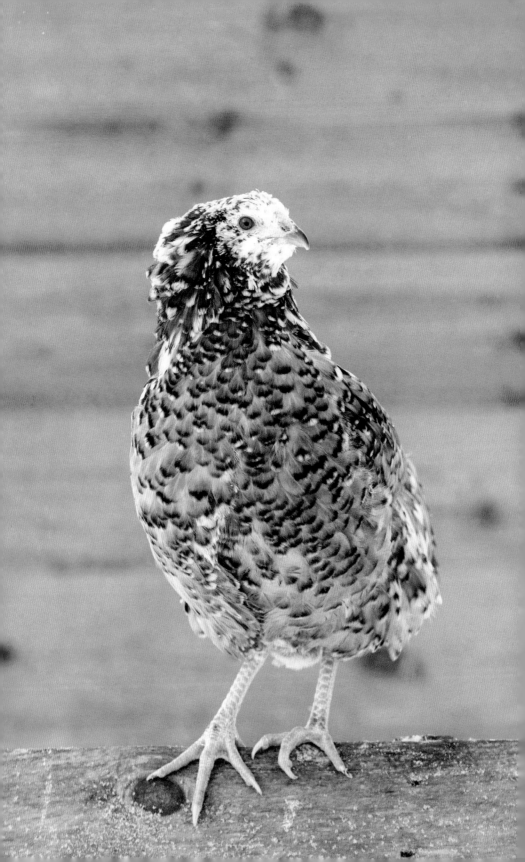

ORIENTAL GAMES

Fanciers contend that Oriental Game Fowl descended from a different, now extinct, ancestor of the Red Junglefowl, which is the ancestor of all other domestic chickens. Genetic studies may help to settle this question. Whether another species lurks in the family tree that has brought Oriental Game Fowl to the present day or not, they are distinctive birds. They share beetle brows, which protect their eyes, strong necks, and *S*-shaped bodies with flat breasts. They are tall and look mean. Oriental breed hens are usually good brooders and mothers, including Phoenix, Yokohama, and Cubalaya breeds. Their short, hard feathers limit the number of eggs they can cover, though.

Malays and Sumatras were included in the original 1874 APA Standard. Cubalayas followed in 1939, and Phoenix in 1965. In 1981, Yokohamas, Aseels, and Shamos were recognized. Additional color varieties of the others were admitted over the years. Fanciers also raise many other Oriental Games. Both the APA and ABA now recognize the Ko Shamo, a true bantam. Russian Orloffs are game in type, descended from Malays and Aseels.

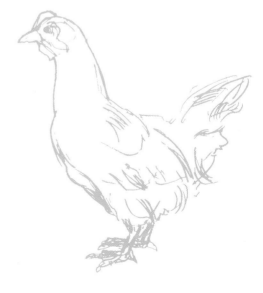

This Russian Orloff hen stays warm in winter under her spangled feathers. Her small comb won't freeze, even in icy weather, but the hen house should have some source of heat. She'll need fresh water to drink.
Paulette Johnson/Fox Hill Photo

MALAY

These tall chickens have a distinctive silhouette with three curves: the neck, the back, and the tail. They have a small pea or strawberry comb. The Malay is one of the oldest chicken breeds. They are well known across North India, Indonesia, and the Malay Peninsula, from which they take their name. They are said to still exist in the wild in northern Malaysia. They were brought to England and from there to America in the nineteenth century.

It's certainly the tallest breed, at more than thirty inches. In the past, Malays were even taller, up to thirty-five inches tall. They are giants among chickens. In the past, Malays weighing over sixteen pounds were documented. Standard weight for large fowl Malay roosters is now nine pounds. Even bantams are among the largest of the small, at forty-four ounces, nearly three pounds. This makes some Malay bantams as large as small full-size chickens. Breeders have added Malays, with their strength, size, and vitality, to their breeding flocks of other breeds to add their desirable traits to the mix.

Many find them good layers of light brown eggs. Their strong, broad head and heavy brows shade eyes with a sharp glint. They look mean and fierce.

The first Malays recognized were the Black-Breasted Red color pattern, the typical colorful chicken color, in 1883. Since then, other colors have been recognized.

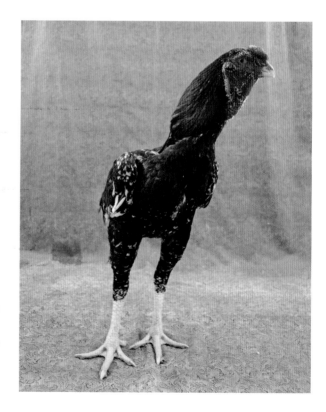

The Oriental Games of Asia have long histories. This Malay is a tall, distinctive bird, with a no-nonsense look in his eye. Malays have so many fine qualities of size, hardiness, and vigor that they have been bred in to many other breeds over the years. *Courtesy of the Livestock Conservancy*

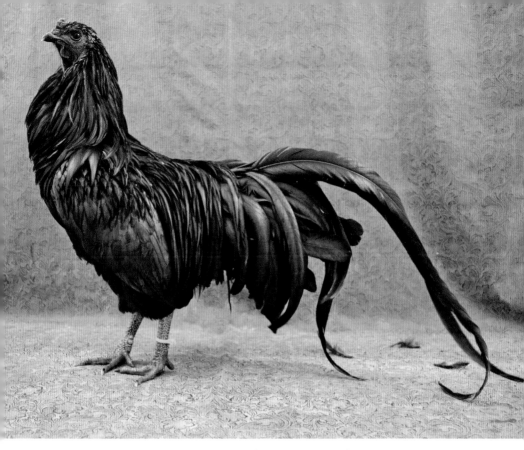

This Sumatra rooster's flowing tail sets him apart from the everyday chicken. Watch his feathers gleam greenish-black in the sun as he struts across the yard. *Courtesy of the Livestock Conservancy*

SUMATRA

The long, black tails of these small chickens identify them as Sumatras.

Sumatras are a long-tailed breed, with the males especially exhibiting long flowing feathers that may drape onto the ground. They are known for their gleaming black feathers, with an iridescent green "beetle" sheen. They have small pea combs and brown eyes set in mulberry or plum-colored skin on their faces, called gypsy coloration. Their multiple spurs, a defect in other breeds, are desirable on Sumatras. Black is the most common color, with blue large fowl and both blue and white bantams also recognized.

Although they come from a very aggressive background known for great fighting spirit, Sumatras are now tame although active birds. They are small and fly well, using their powerful wings to take off vertically.

They are a landrace originally from the island of Sumatra in western Indonesia. The first trio was brought to the United States in 1847, shipped directly to Boston from Angers Points on the island. There, they were bred with local American game fowl.

They lay well, white or lightly tinted eggs, making them an exception to the rule of thumb that birds with dark earlobes lay brown eggs.

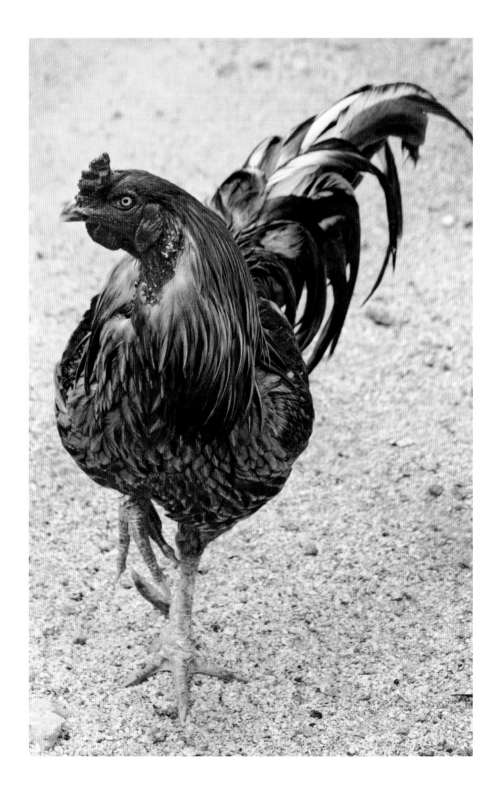

CUBALAYA

Cubalayas stand upright, the feathers of their back and tail descending to the ground in a sweeping line. The long, wide tail divides down the middle to earn the description "lobster tail." Sickles and coverts often drag on the ground.

They usually have small dome-like multiple spurs. In most breeds, this is a serious defect, but in Cubalayas, it's desirable. The Cubalaya is considered the national breed of Cuba, but is virtually identical to some of the Pheasant Malay type fowls of the Philippines and Southeast Asia. The only difference of note would be the uniform white leg color and uniform pea combs of the Cubalaya. Reportedly, some western game blood was infused into the Cubalaya, but it influenced color pattern development more than type. Pea-combed Malays of the tall bodied type and Shamos or Thai Games have also been used to increase size in the Cubalaya, which may have since declined due to inbreeding. However, in both cases the original type was maintained.

Spanish sailors brought Asian game fowl to Cuba from the Philippines in the mid-nineteenth century. Cuban development of the breed stressed exhibition qualities but never lost sight of their utility for production of both meat and eggs.

At six pounds for a mature rooster and four pounds for a hen, their fine-grained white flesh is good eating, and they are respectable layers of white eggs. They share with other game breeds their hardiness and resistance to disease. Hens are good setters and mothers. Breeders report high fertility rates.

The APA recognizes three color varieties: Black-Breasted Red, White, and Black. As with other games, fanciers raise many other colors, such as Silver Duckwing and Golden Duckwing. The Cenizos is ash-colored; the Indios Cenizos is ash-colored breasted red. If you intend your Cubalayas for showing, hatch early, because it takes time for the males to grow a full tail and for the pullets to gain weight.

Experienced breeder Horst Schmudde finds they nearly nourish themselves when kept on sufficient free range. With a fierce protective temperament, the Cubalaya is well able to fend for itself, but it needs space from other birds.

Despite a somewhat fierce look, they are gentle and friendly with people. Breeders who spend time with their birds may find they have a rooster on one knee and a hen on the other, looking to be petted.

This Cubalaya, from Cuba, indicates his fighting heritage with the spurs on the back of his legs. Multiple spurs are a defect in other breeds, but they are desirable in Cubalayas. *Mauro Rodrigues/ Getty Images*

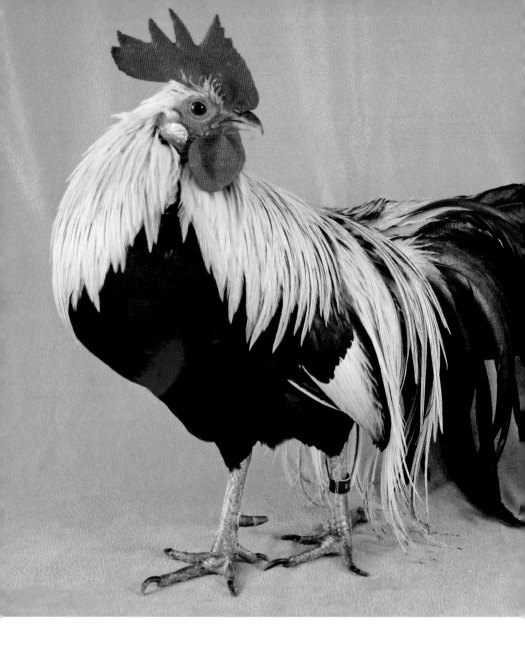

PHOENIX AND OTHER LONG-TAILED BREEDS

The long tails on Phoenix chickens distinguish them. Their tail, sickle, and saddle feathers are longer (up to five feet!) and there are more of them than any other recognized breed.

Phoenix chickens were bred from Japanese Onigadori chickens, which have long, flowing tail feathers. When Onigadori chickens came to Europe in the nineteenth century, the birds were not strong. Breeders who wanted to maintain birds with such beautiful feathers crossed them with Leghorns and other games such as Malays, Old English, and Modern Games to make

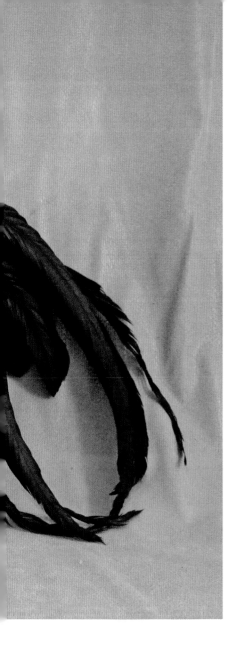

Phoenix are more resilient than their forebears, because they get new feathers more often. They grow rigid sickle feathers two to five feet long, enhanced by saddle feathers twelve to eighteen inches long and coverts dragging on the ground. Nevertheless, keeping roosters of this breed in top condition requires special feather care and a higher protein diet (meal worms and fish products can help). They need perches high enough so that the feathers can't drag on the ground, and clean bedding such as wood shavings, no mud or sand. The hens are good layers and, like other Games, good mothers.

In Japan, the Onigadori breed is designated as a special natural monument, and five of the others—Shokoku, Ohiki, Kashiwa, Satsumadori, and Minohiki— are natural monument fowl breeds. Taking eggs out of Japan is prohibited, so American long-tailed chickens are descended from birds that were brought here in the past. Long tailed chickens are also popular in Germany and other European countries. Phoenix is the only long-tailed breed recognized by the APA and ABA, in several color varieties.

Onigadori and other long-tailed breeds raised in Japan are confined to Tombako, meaning rooster stop boxes. The chicken lives a limited life, confined to a perch and taken out for walks, with a keeper following holding up the tail feathers on a frame. You won't see that in an American backyard.

them hardier. The result is the Phoenix, rising from the ashes of a sickly breed.

Onigadori are able to grow tail feathers over twenty feet long, because they have a recessive gene that limits molting to every three years or even longer. That gives the feathers more time to grow. Phoenix molt every year or two.

YOKOHAMA

These graceful game chickens, white with red shoulders and breast feathers, are Yokohamas. They are the only breed with the Red Shoulder color pattern. This unusual pattern of red shoulders and red breast with white flecks, under a cape of white flowing feathers is dramatic. The flowing hackle feathers may form a full circle around the neck. This color pattern was imported to the United States in the 1970s. Solid white Yokohamas are also recognized, as are Dark Brown, Light Brown, and Silver bantams.

The Yokohama breed got its name from the port from which they were shipped to Paris back in 1864. The birds were Japanese Minohikis, but over time Yokohamas have been bred with other Games to develop unique qualities that make them a separate breed. Yokohamas are considered a German creation from Japanese ancestry.

Yokohamas are Oriental Games, carrying themselves with high station but more horizontal than their tall Game relatives. They have no wattles or only very small ones. Yokohamas have walnut combs. These elegant birds are more decorative than productive, but the hens lay white eggs and, like other Games, are good mothers.

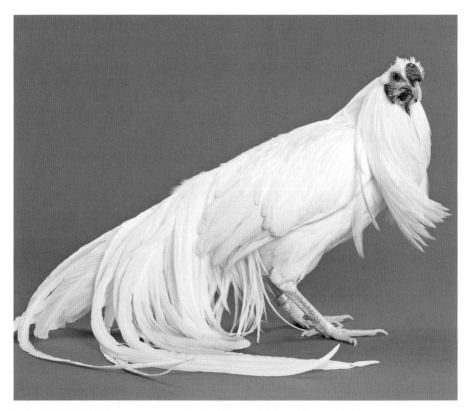

This solid white Yokohama rooster carries the history of Oriental Games in his heritage. His walnut comb results from both rose and pea comb genes, furrowed like half a walnut. *Derek Sasaki/www.mypetchicken.com*

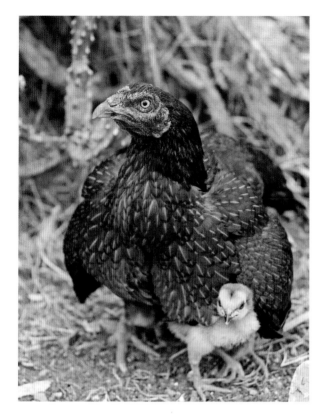

This Aseel mother takes good care of her chicks. Like other Oriental Game breeds, she is a good brooder. She will protect her chicks from danger while teaching the basics of what to eat and how to survive in the flock. *thinkdo/Shutterstock*

ASEEL

These tall, imposing chickens look like the fighting chickens they are. Their bodies are strong and heavily muscled, set off by the short, tight-fitting feathers. They are Aseels, forebears of today's Cornish, the stocky bird that, as a hybrid with Plymouth Rocks, is America's meat bird.

The breed's history dates back as far as 3,500 years and is so intertwined with the Malay and Shamo that it's unclear which was the progenitor. Pakistan and India are its original home, and in India, Aseel is the general word for all game fowl.

Aseels were expressly bred for cock fighting. The Rajahs of Oudh, a northwestern province of India, kept detailed stud books of their fighting birds thousands of years ago.

They were first admitted to the Standard in 1981, as Oriental Games acquired more followers in the United States. Black-Breasted Red, Dark, Spangled, White, and Wheaten female varieties are recognized. Fanciers classify them in three sizes, from fifteen pound roosters over twenty-nine inches tall to small ones weighing less than five pounds standing less than twenty inches tall.

They are known for their aggressive disposition and willingness to pick a fight and require special care in keeping them in separate pens.

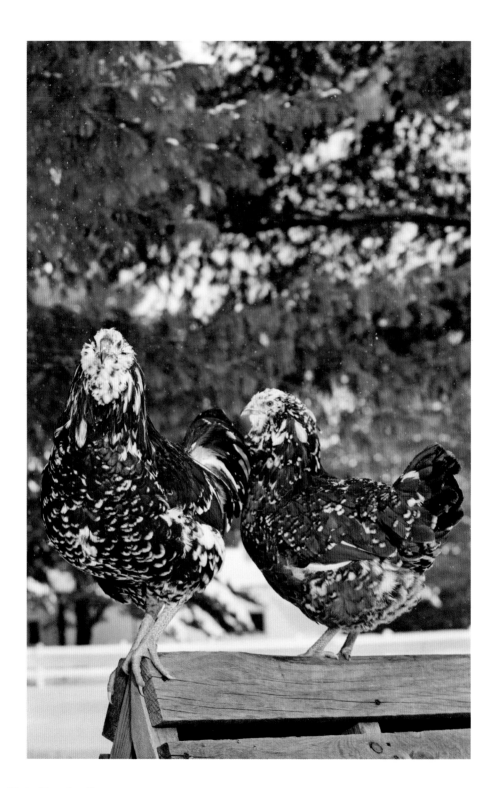

ORLOFF

Russian Orloffs have an expression often described as "gloomy" and "vindictive." A feathery scarf surrounds its neck, and a small comb sits on top of the head, above feathery eyebrows. Earlobes and wattles are completely covered by feathers.

Their walnut combs, which may have a few hair-like feathers springing from them, don't freeze in cold weather. Their wattles and earlobes are small and also unaffected by cold. As befits a bird adapted to the Russian climate, these birds are hardy.

They originated in northern Iran's Gilan province and share an Asian Game appearance, with their long, strong Malay legs like the local chickens of Iran, Afghanistan, and Pakistan.

In Iran, the breed was called the Chilianskaia. In the late nineteenth century, Russian nobleman Count Orloff Techesmensky brought some to Moscow, where they became known by his name. In the 1920s, another Prince Orloff, living in exile from the Revolution in England, acquired some Orloff chickens and won some poultry show prizes with them, keeping up the family name and tradition.

Russian Orloffs were included in the APA Standard from 1876 through 1888 but were dropped from later Standards. Bantams are still included in the ABA Standard, but they are not often seen.

The Spangled variety is most likely to be seen in the United States, but breeders in Germany and England raise other colors that American backyarders might keep, including White, Mahogany, Black-Breasted Red, and others. Their feathery faces and short, hooked beaks distinguish this breed's appearance from any other.

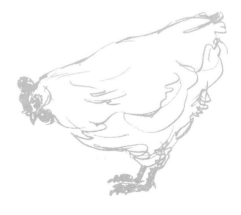

Russian Orloff chickens are rare but beautiful. Their small combs resist freezing in sub-zero temperatures. Their spangled plumage is especially thick and helps these hardy chickens survive harsh weather. *Paulette Johnson/Fox Hill Photo*

SHAMO

Shamos almost look part hawk. They carry muscular bodies on long legs. Feathers are tight and smooth, but in places they hardly cover the bird, leaving patches of skin showing.

Shamos were developed in Japan from Thai Games, beginning in the seventeenth century early Tokugawa period of active Southeast Asian trade. Their meat became popular as "pep food" and was recommended for sumo wrestlers. Shamo means "fighter."

After cockfighting was outlawed in Japan in 1924, they were bred for exhibition. They have always been docile with people and are now protected by law in Japan, along with other important breeds, for their historic significance. After World War II, American soldiers brought Shamos back with them from Japan.

Japanese breeders have developed many variations in four size categories, from two pounds to twelve. Shamos shown in the United States reflect their Thai Game heritage. They are tall, imperious, even described as having a cruel look, like a bird of prey. Roosters can stand over two feet tall. They are closely related to Malays but have shorter legs and are shorter overall.

Large fowl can be shown at up to eleven pounds for roosters, seven for hens, but breeders may raise larger birds. Fanciers breed many other varieties beyond the four recognized ones.

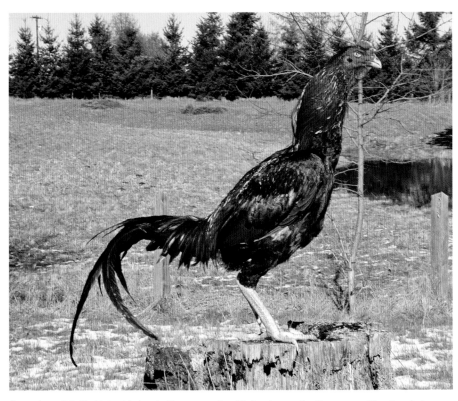

Snow doesn't intimidate this hardy Shamo rooster. His hard game feathers cover him closely to keep him warm. This one looks like he is ready to stretch out and crow! *Courtesy of Fort Bantam*

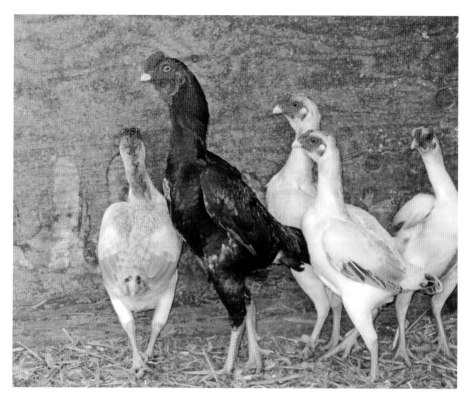

This Ko Shamo rooster and his hens show the typical body type of three equal parts: one-third head and neck, one-third body, and one-third leg. He may stand so tall that he walks on his front toes. *Walt Leonard*

KO SHAMO

Ko Shamos are small but have the powerful frame of Oriental game fowl. Their combs sit above their beaks like crumpled flowers, fierce eyes standing atop a neck stretched to full height. Their feathers mold closely to their muscular bodies. Some even have bare spots on their necks and breasts.

The Ko Shamo is a true bantam, not related to the large fowl Shamo. They trace their ancestry to Siam, where game fowl have been raised for centuries. The Ko Shamo traces its history back to sixteenth century Japanese traders in Southeast Asia and India.

The ABA gave it recognition in 2013. The official standard describes the Ko Shamo as having "a cocky attitude, upright stance, prominent shoulders." Ko Shamos have a chrysanthemum comb, a gnarly red crown. Smaller pea and walnut combs are acceptable on large fowl Shamos.

Ko Shamos are required to have split wings, which means a feather is permanently missing, leaving a gap between the primary and secondary wing feathers. In any other breed, this is a defect serious enough to disqualify a bird from being judged at a show. In Ko Shamos, it is a distinctive identifying trait.

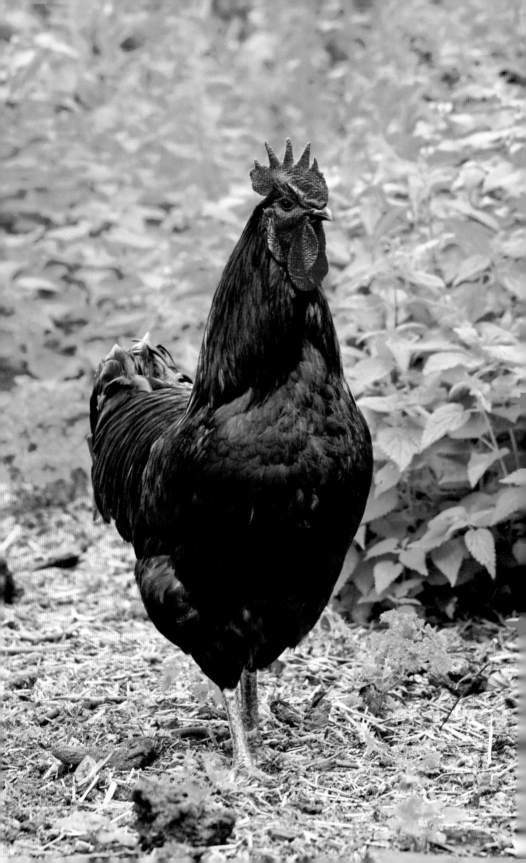

AMERICAN BREEDS

All breeds raised in America reflect unique local climates and regional and national styles. The American breeds, as classified by the APA, are breeds that have American history that distinguishes them from others. They have all developed regional characteristics that distinguish local conditions and their breeders' preferences.

When most Americans lived on farms, chickens were part of the livestock that kept the farm going. American breeds were *general-purpose* chickens, all-around solid breeds that contributed to farm success. That term fell out of use in the 1930s, as commercial farms began focusing on increased production. It was replaced by the term *dual-purpose*, breeds that were raised to gain weight faster and lay more eggs sooner. Dual-purpose and general-purpose are now used interchangeably, although there's a nuance of difference to the advanced chicken keeper.

The American background is obvious in their names: Plymouth Rock, Wyandotte, Rhode Island Red and White, Buckeye, Jersey Giant, New Hampshire, and Delaware. Others are confusing: Dominiques and Chanteclers sound French, Javas seem South Asian, Hollands imply European. Lamonas are named after the man who developed them. They all reflect America's heritage as a melting pot for immigrants from around the world.

Lamonas and Hollands are extremely rare. One breeder is re-creating the Lamona, and a few are raising Hollands. Both breeds are twentieth-century composite breeds, created for commercial flocks. They remain recognized by the Standard of Perfection, but casual observers are unlikely ever to encounter one.

Commercial hatcheries have stepped up to offer backyard chicken owners production birds. As hybrids, they will not reproduce themselves. Most backyarders aren't breeding their birds, so hybrids can fulfill their desire for chickens and fresh eggs. Hybrids such as sex-links and production reds are distinctly American. Commercial marketing departments give them flashy names such as Red Star and Cinnamon Queen.

The biggest chickens in the backyard are the Jersey Giants. This chicken could herald a return of the roast chicken for a feast. Hens lay big, brown eggs. *Cornelia Pithart/Shutterstock*

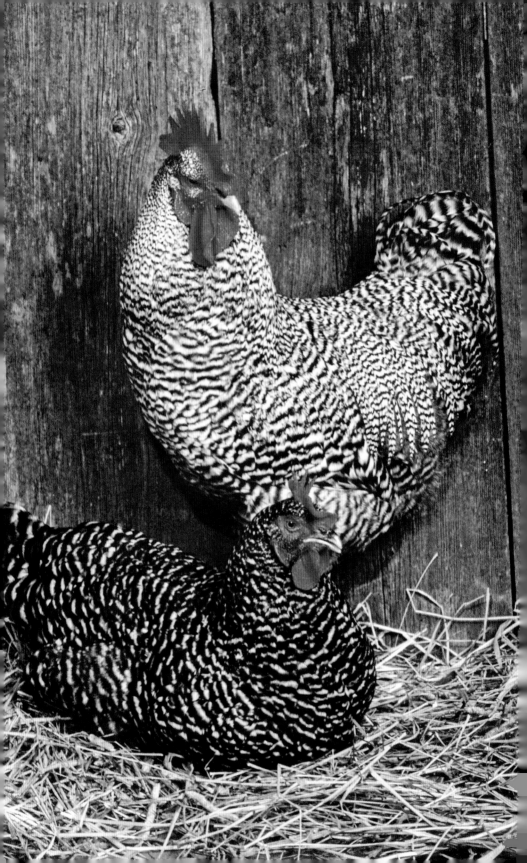

PLYMOUTH ROCK

Plymouth Rocks are the first breed listed in the APA Standard. The barred variety, meaning the alternating dark and light lines on the feathers, was the first recognized in the 1874 original and remains the best known. You'll often hear them called simply Barred Rocks.

Recognize Plymouth Rocks by their shape, size, and single combs. Dominiques have similar black and white barred feathers, but have rose combs and are smaller. The Rock shape is the most important quality: a broad, level back, four inches or more between the nape of the neck and the beginning of the tail, then rising with a slight concave sweep to the tail. Broad shoulders and strong tail feathers well spread, carried moderately upright, "build up the back to the proper ending," according to *The Poultry Book* from 1912. They are hefty birds, at nine and a half pounds for roosters and seven and a half pounds for hens.

Like all American breeds, they have yellow skin. This comes from the Cochins that were bred into them in the nineteenth century. That barred feather pattern is crisp and clear, bright rather than smoky. Each feather should be barred all the way down to the base of the quill. Plymouth Rocks are useful, active, dual-purpose birds that have attracted many followers over the years. Their eggs range from lightly tinted to dark brown. Frank Reese of Good Shepherd Poultry Ranch in Lindsborg, Kansas, considers it "the perfect bird for outdoor production," along with New Hampshires.

Their admiring breeders have developed six additional varieties recognized by the Standard: White, Buff, Silver Penciled, Partridge, Columbian, and Blue. Bantams are also recognized in Black. Combs should have five points, but the small size of bantams makes four points acceptable. Four points may even be nicely symmetrical.

Plymouth Rocks were developed in Massachusetts after the Civil War and named for one of the state's most famous landmarks. Joseph Spaulding of Putnam, Connecticut, began the breed by crossing a single-comb Dominique male on a Black Cochin (at that time, the clean-legged Shanghae), and others later added Minorca, White Cochin, Black Spanish, Gray Dorking, Buff Cochin, and others. They were originally shown in the Dorking class, which has since been subsumed in the American class. Dorkings are now shown in the English class.

Plymouth Rock chickens are named for one of the most famous features in Massachusetts. There are many color varieties. These are Barred. You will often hear them called simply Barred Rocks.
Paulette Johnson/Fox Hill Photo

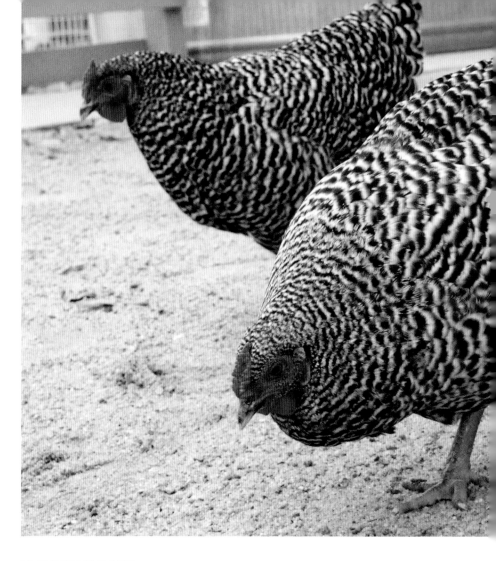

DOMINIQUE

Dominiques are recognized by their black-and-white barred feathers and small classic rose comb, with an upturned spike at the back. Don't confuse them with Barred Plymouth Rocks, which have similar feathers but a single comb.

Dominiques are considered the first American breed. Their French-sounding name comes from the idea that they came from birds brought to America from Santo Domingo in the Caribbean. Maybe it happened that way, or maybe not. Although their origins are clouded in history, they were plentiful in the United States by 1820 and were documented on Ohio farms by 1850.

By 1890, the Barred Plymouth Rock had replaced the Dominique on many farms. Dominiques were eclipsed by Rocks in the early twentieth century and nearly disappeared with the rise of industrial poultry methods by mid-century. Dominiques rallied in the late twentieth century under the influence of significant breeders but have since struggled.

Their feathers are barred, ideally silver white and dove-gray, in the color pattern known in other breeds as cuckoo. The

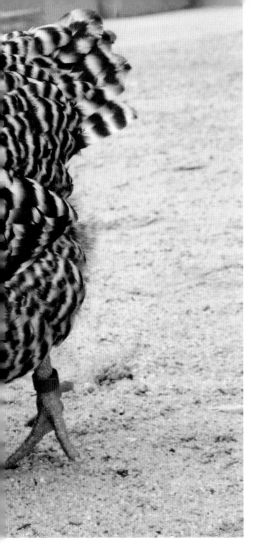

Where the name "Dominique" came from is lost in history, but they are the first recognized American breed. You may have heard them called Dominickers. *Courtesy of the Livestock Conservancy*

colors blur as one watches them, making them look blue. That color pattern may have provided protective camouflage for them when they found their own living by foraging in the barnyard. Dominiques are still good foragers.

The males have longer sickle feathers. Their bright yellow legs stand out. Getting the rose comb perfect is a challenge to breeders. It may lack the required spike or the spike may be misshapen. Tail angle in both males and females can be difficult to perfect. Dominique tails should stand at a jaunty 45-degree angle.

Dominiques are a general-purpose barnyard breed. They make good roasters or fryers at seven pounds for mature cocks and five pounds for mature hens. They are steady, reliable layers of brown eggs. The hens will settle in and brood eggs and raise the chicks they hatch.

They strut around their yard with head held high on arched neck. The roosters hold their heads up so well, their backs have a *U*-shaped silhouette. They hold their full tails higher than other American breeds.

WYANDOTTE

A Wyandotte's distinctive silhouette is created by its smooth broad feathers and close-fitting plumage. Even the rose comb curves around the head, fitting neatly and closely, rather than having its spike stand out. It is a bird of circle curves, from its rose comb and head to its well-rounded breast.

Wyandottes were developed in the post–Civil War era, possibly with the goal of developing an improved Cochin bantam. Because the cross breeding resulted in large, meaty birds that laid well, the birds were in demand. Before a breed description was defined in the Standard, breeders displayed and sold whatever birds they had.

Another cold-hardy breed, Wyandottes lay eggs ranging in color from light to rich brown. That distinctive rose comb, probably inherited from their Spangled Hamburg forebears, is resistant to freezing. Dark and Light Brahmas gave them size and color pattern, although the Dark Brahma color markings are unacceptable in the breed now.

It's an excellent dual-purpose breed for the small flock owner and exhibition poultry keeper. They are substantial birds, with excellent meat. Hens lay around 200 eggs a year, with some reports of as many as 240.

Wyandottes are mentioned as early as 1873, but were not admitted to the APA Standard of Perfection until 1883, when the Silver Laced variety was the first admitted. The Silver Laced large fowl has the color and pattern of Silver Sebright bantams.

Wisconsin breeders developed Golden Laced Wyandottes from a Partridge Cochin/Brown Leghorn cross rooster and a Silver Laced Wyandotte hen. They were admitted to the Standard in 1888, along with the Whites. The White variety was selectively bred from sports (chicks that are a different color from the parents)

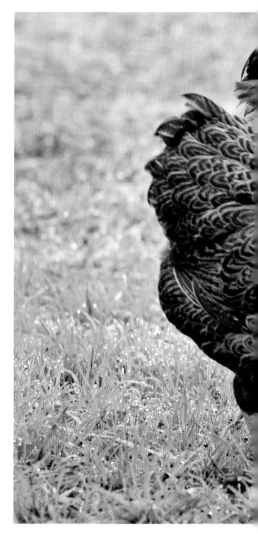

that appeared spontaneously in Silver Laced flocks. At first, the white sports were considered an embarrassment, an indication of lack of purity in the flock.

As Wyandottes gained popularity, their advocates developed Buff, Black, Partridge, Columbian, and Blue varieties, which are now recognized, in addition to the Silver Laced, Golden Laced, Silver Penciled, and White varieties. Fanciers raise Cuckoo, Buff Laced, Violet Laced,

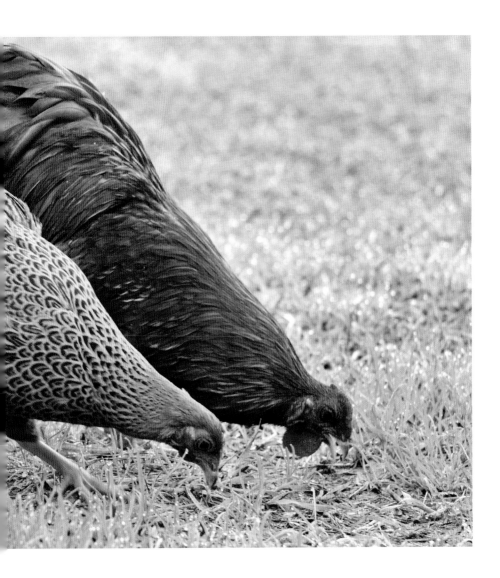

Red, Blue Laced Red, Buff Columbian, and other unrecognized varieties. Bantams are also recognized in Barred, Birchen, Black-Breasted Red, Blue Red, Brown Red, Buff Columbian, Lemon Blue, Splash, and White Laced Red.

The Columbian color pattern that now graces varieties of many breeds got its name from the Wyandottes exhibited at the 1893 Columbian Exposition, the World's Fair, in Chicago.

This pair of Wyandottes is an unusual chocolate partridge color pattern. Wyandottes are a classic dual-purpose American breed. In backyards, their well-rounded shape is usually seen in the other nine recognized colors.
Courtesy Greenfire Farms

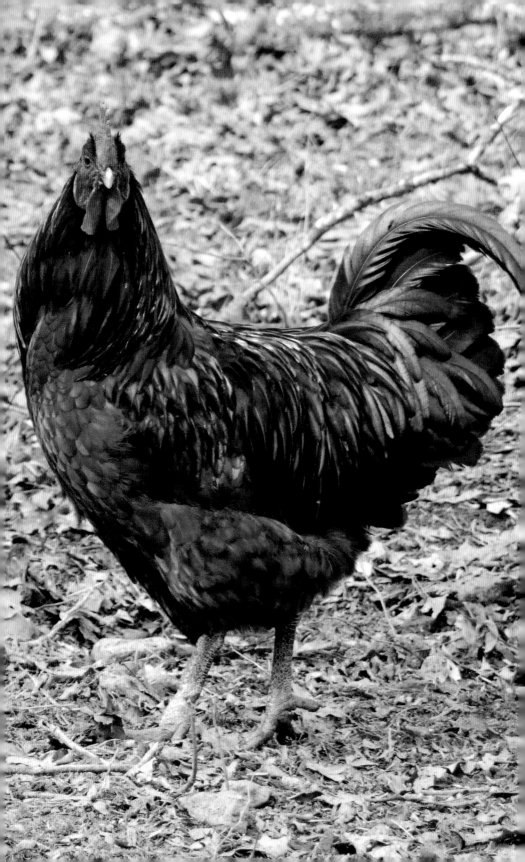

JAVA

Recognize the Java by the way it holds its tail at a jaunty 55-degree angle. The tail's gracefully curved feathers are either solid black or black with white tips, lustrous and glistening green.

The Java is one of the American class foundation breeds, despite taking its name for the island in Indonesia.

Back in the days of sailing ships trading with Asia for spices, the Java arrived in ports along the East Coast, such as New Bedford, Rhode Island. Ship captains brought red Javas and other red chickens, such as Shanghais and Great Malays, along with their cargo in the 1830s. By 1883, only Black and Mottled varieties were admitted to the American Poultry Association's Standard of Perfection.

The Java became popular as a high-class market fowl. Its fine qualities were bred into flocks that became the Black Jersey Giant and the Barred Plymouth Rock. The breed nearly disappeared by the end of the twentieth century, but recently attention from specialty breeders and historical societies such as the Garfield Farm Museum in Illinois has given the breed a second chance.

The Java grows slowly, putting weight on its bones and maturing its feathers over months rather than weeks. It is an excellent forager, happy finding its living among the shrubs and bushes. It's a fast runner, able to escape predators on its feet.

Javas are an example of the unseen genetic mix concealed under their black, or mottled black and white, feathers.

Because the genes are so pervasive, some breeders keep two flocks, one black and one mottled. Then, the birds can be assigned to the appropriate flock as their plumage grows. Both feather colors are acceptable.

The APA Standard of Perfection describes the Mottled Java's white-tipped feather pattern and "broken" leaden blue and yellow leg color. Black Javas have black or nearly black legs, but with yellow on the bottom of their feet. The Auburn variety, a color not recognized by any Standard, disappeared in the nineteenth century, but some Auburn chicks were hatched in an Illinois breeding project in 2004. The color's unexpected appearance tantalizes breeders with a hint of what other genes might be concealed in our flocks.

The Java is a foundation American breed, honoring its origins in Southeast Asia with its name. Javas weren't suited to industrial chicken keeping, but their proud spirit and beautiful black feathers won breeders' and historians' hearts. *Courtesy of the Livestock Conservancy*

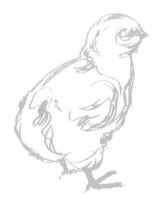

RHODE ISLAND RED AND WHITE

Rhode Island Reds (RIRs) are American icons. Even Rhode Island Red aficionados find it difficult to express the subtle beauty of the Rhode Island Red's feathers.

When your eye has learned the horizontal oblong body shape of the Red, you will be able to recognize the distinctive appearance of the White. Reds may have either single comb or rose comb. Whites have rose combs.

RIRs are slightly smaller and brighter red than the Buckeye, which was also being developed at the turn of the twentieth century.

Rhode Island Reds remain one of the most popular breeds, for small and for commercial laying flocks. RIRs are the source of commercial brown eggs. The industrial birds are smaller, lighter, and less inclined to become broody. They would not meet the Standard of Perfection required by poultry judges.

Production RIRs can lay up to 300 eggs a year. Exhibition birds that meet the APA Standard will lay fewer eggs but can be shown at poultry shows.

RIRs were developed in Rhode Island and Massachusetts in the mid-nineteenth century as a dual-purpose farm and commercial breed. Red Malay Game and Red Cochin China roosters arrived on sailing ships in the seaport towns of Little Compton, Rhode Island, and Westport, Massachusetts. Sea captains sold them to local farmers, who bred them into their flocks. Auburn Javas also arrived on those boats, contributing their rectangular body. Rose-Comb Brown Leghorns added to the mix to produce the "hardy red cock of a type that showed vigor" that was traditional in New England utility flocks of the second half of the nineteenth century, according to Dr. N. B. Aldrich of Massachusetts and W. J. Drisko, secretary of the Rhode Island Red Club in 1912.

In 1904 the single comb variety was recognized, followed by the rose comb in 1905. A pea comb variety was raised, but lost favor as not having good type or vigor. The original description of the plumage in the 1905 Standard was "rich, brilliant red." The current Standard calls for "lustrous, rich, dark red." These refinements are the kind of subtlety that only experience and working with poultry masters can confer.

Today, Rhode Island Reds remain one of the most popular breeds, both as large fowl and as bantams.

The Rhode Island Red is popular in backyards and on exhibition and are honored for their beauty as well as their egg laying. *Paulette Johnson/ Fox Hill Photo*

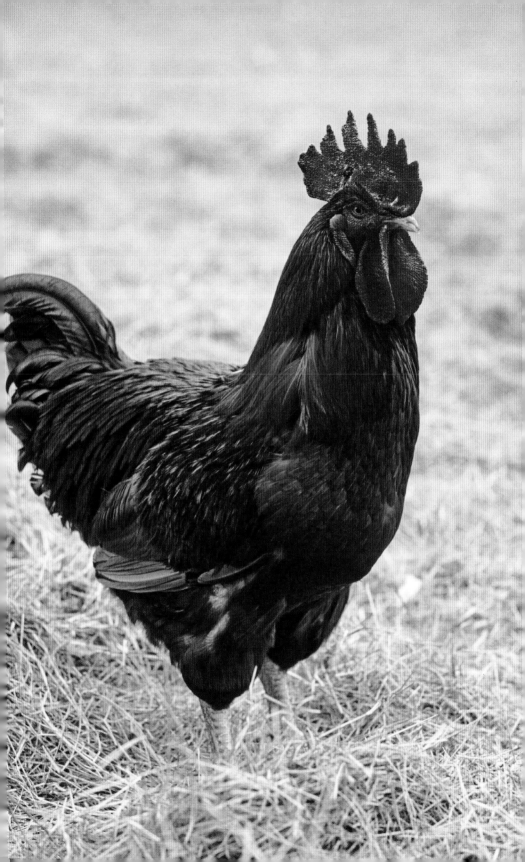

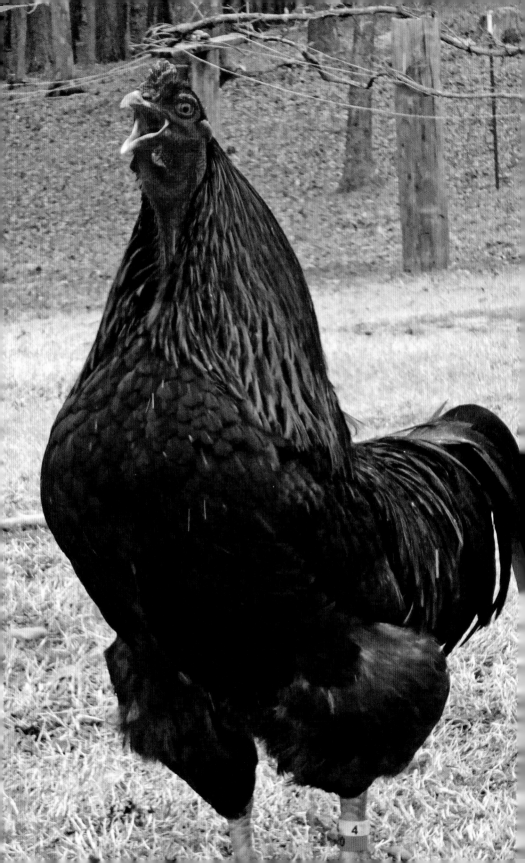

BUCKEYE

A buckeye is a nut produced by the tree of the same name. It gives its name to the state of Ohio. That's where the Buckeye chicken breed was developed. Recognize them by their glossy reddish brown feathers.

No chicken breed is perfect, but many Buckeye breeders figure they have come close with this breed. Buckeyes are friendly and easy-going, with excellent vigor, resilience, and disease resistance in a bird that grows to a solid size and lays plenty of eggs. They have played an interesting role in poultry history, giving their breeders the honor of carrying the torch into the future.

One of the Buckeye's distinctions is that it is the only breed credited entirely to a woman for its creation. The estimable Nettie Metcalf created the breed at the turn of the twentieth century. She was intrigued with the Rhode Island Red, even calling her birds Buckeye Reds when she first introduced them, as a pea comb variety, distinct from the single and rose comb varieties of Rhode Island Reds.

Her birds' darker mahogany color and separate breeding gave the Buckeye a distinct identity, and she observed that they might well be confused with the RIR and absorbed into that breed unless efforts were made to keep them separate.

Her first cross, Buff Cochin cockerels on Barred Rock hens, "produced a big, lazy fowl, so I looked around for something else to mix in." She settled on Black-Breasted Red Games and selected the red offspring from that mating and bred them to each other. Her full account is reprinted on the website of the American Buckeye Club.

"My, what a flock I raised that year," she remembered. "No wonder my friends laughed. Green legs and feathered legs, buff chicks, black chicks, and even red-and-black barred chicks; single combs and pea combs and no combs at all, but all fighters from away back."

Although Cornish birds were not included in Metcalf's original breeding, the Games she used would likely have had Cornish in their background. Buckeye heads have a particularly Cornish shape. Their pea combs come from their Cornish side.

Relations among birds are congenial, with roosters taking a gentle interest in watching over the flock and little fighting between males. Their social nature is expressed in a variety of vocalizations, from a purr to a roar, particularly among the roosters.

Ohio takes pride in the Buckeye! That signature deep, rich red plumage inspired the name of this cold-hardy, dual-purpose breed. This rooster presides over hens that lay well even in winter.
Christopher McCary

CHANTECLER

Identify Chanteclers by their small cushion combs and small, well-rounded wattles. If the owner is nearby and can catch one for you, squeeze their plumage. Their feathers are tight, but the downy undercoat insulates them from the cold.

Chanteclers were developed as a distinctive Canadian breed by Canadian monk Brother Wilfred Chatelain. The breed was admitted to the American Standard in 1921. They thrive in cold weather. Their distinctive small comb and wattles resist freezing, and the extra feathering keeps them warm. Chanteclers are sociable and charming. They can be shy with strangers but when socialized, have even been used as therapy hens.

Chanteclers manage happily on the snow. They are alert and active. They'll call out any visitors or dangers in the vicinity. They are good foragers, content to explore the shady cool sections that other breeds ignore in favor of warmer, sunnier locations.

They are good winter layers of brown eggs, continuing despite cold temperatures and declining sunlight. Their meat is delicious, and they can be butchered young, for a smaller bird, or allowed time to grow larger.

Although Chanteclers adapt to confinement, crowded indoor conditions are too warm for their cold-hardy constitution. Keeping them in warmer climates affects their cold-adapted traits. If it's warm, they don't need those downy feathers. Warmer temperatures, whether natural or artificially provided to increase laying, will inevitably lead to birds that are adapted to those warmer conditions.

The Chantecler's demise was heavily publicized in 1979 and 1980, but while there were no Chanteclers at universities or commercial hatcheries, small flock owners still had them.

With the precise records that Brother Wilfred kept, it's also been possible to re-create Chanteclers. It's unclear now whether any Chanteclers being shown today are descended from the original birds or have been re-created.

Brother Wilfred's original Chanteclers were white. The Partridge color variety was developed from an entirely different lineage by Dr. John E. Wilkinson in 1919, resulting in black, white, red, buff, and Columbian varieties.

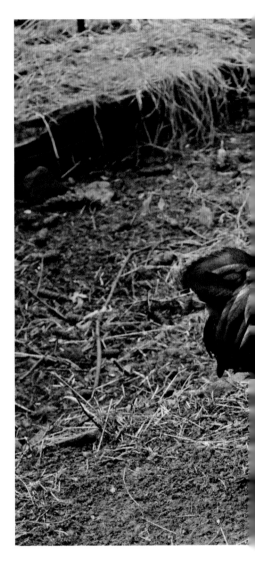

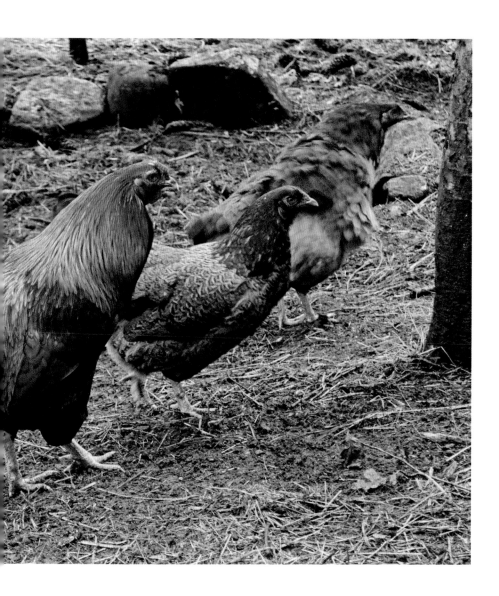

He applied for APA recognition of his birds as a separate breed, but the APA recognized the Partridge variety in 1935 as a color variety of Chanteclers. Chanteclers are also raised in bantam varieties, which were developed later.

However, the White Chanteclers remain distinct from the Partridge and Buff varieties. Original White Chanteclers have longer backs and harder feathers than the color varieties. Buff Chanteclers are not yet recognized.

This Partridge Chantecler rooster has the cushion comb that suits the cold weather of Canadian winters since small combs resist freezing. His colored plumage helps camouflage him as he forages in the bushes. *Courtesy of the Livestock Conservancy*

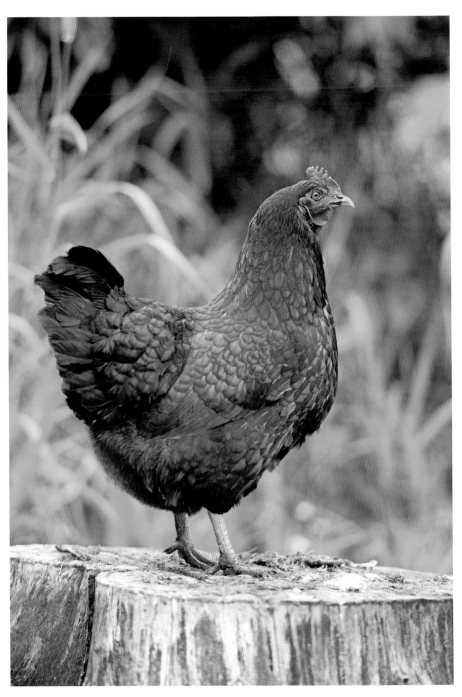

The largest American breed, Jersey Giant hens like this one weigh ten pounds, larger than roosters of most other breeds. They lay plenty of dark brown eggs too. *Anna Hoychuk/Shutterstock*

JERSEY GIANT

Recognize Jersey Giants by—you guessed it—size. At thirteen pounds and two feet tall, Jersey Giant roosters live up to their name. Hens, at ten pounds and a foot and a half tall, are bigger than roosters of most other breeds.

Most Jersey Giants are black, the original color developed by the brothers Black, John and Thomas, of New Jersey back in the 1890s. They sold poultry to the city-dwellers of New York and Philadelphia, who wanted big roasting chickens. The Black brothers' idea was to create a chicken big enough to replace the turkey at holiday feasts.

To create the Giants, the Black brothers crossed Javas with Dark Brahmas and Black Langshans and selected the biggest birds for the next round of breeding. Big, muscular Cornish was probably added along the way. By 1895, their flock had the largest birds. They were mostly black, so they came to be known as Black's Giants. Later, in 1917, another breeder suggested honoring the state where they were developed by calling them Jersey Giants. The breed was accepted into the Standard in 1922.

Because they need more time to grow to achieve their larger size, their meat requires longer roasting. They are not recommended as fryers or broilers. Despite their large size, they are also good layers of large and extra-large brown eggs.

Jersey Giants that are caponized, castrated like steers, grow faster and bigger. Jersey Giant capons could be as large as ten or twelve pounds by seven months old. Caponizing is rarely done today, but it could be a market niche for a small producer.

Like the Javas, Giants have yellow skin. White sports were bred to create a white variety, which was recognized by the APA in 1947. Both varieties are solid color. Blue Jersey Giants were developed from a white sport bred back to a black male resulting in some chickens with splash plumage. Breeding those splash females to a black male eventually resulted in chickens with blue coloring. The blue color pattern in chickens never breeds 100 percent blue birds. It's called incomplete dominance and results in about a quarter of the offspring growing up black, a quarter growing up splash, and half growing up blue.

Bantams are on the Inactive list. But then, what's the point of a bantam Giant?

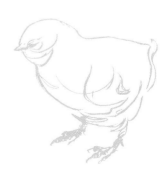

NEW HAMPSHIRE

New Hampshires are the color of a pumpkin, topped off with a black tail. Hens have black ticking on the hackle feathers around their necks. Roosters have darker hackles, without the black edging. New Hampshires have broad, level backs and carry their tails higher than the related Rhode Island Reds. Their tails are not big, but boast beautiful red-edged black feathers shimmering with green. The hens' combs lop over. That lopped comb disqualifies most single comb breeds from competition, but New Hampshire hens are specifically exempted from that rule. The APA gives any single combed hen in or near production allowance on a lopped comb.

In the early nineteenth century, New England farmers liked those red chickens. Local trends led New Hampshire farmers to develop the lighter color, while Rhode Island farmers preferred the darker red. By the twentieth century, breeders in New Hampshire were focused on refining a distinct breed. They aimed for birds that would grow faster than the existing Rhode Island Reds. The other desired characteristics included early maturity, large brown eggs, quick feathering, strength, and vigor.

Selective breeding of individuals excelling in those qualities from around 1915 resulted in the New Hampshire breed. Early feathering may have brought the lighter red color with it. New Hampshires were admitted to the Standard in 1935.

Professor A. W. Richardson, known by his nickname Red, championed development of New Hampshires and focused on the meat and egg production rather than refining the color.

This breed satisfies both meat and egg production goals. They have deep, well-rounded bodies, meaty and strong, and are able to lay about 160 eggs a year. Some strains are bred more for meat production and do not lay as well as the dual-purpose strains. Strains selected for egg production are usually smaller than Standard weight of six and a half pounds for the hens. Roosters should weigh eight and a half pounds for exhibition.

New Hampshires crossed with Barred Rocks contributed to the development of Delawares. That cross is often used to raise broilers and roasting chickens. They lay well and can get big enough, beyond the Standard weight, to be good meat birds.

Bantams are also shown. Both large fowl and bantams make excellent backyard chickens.

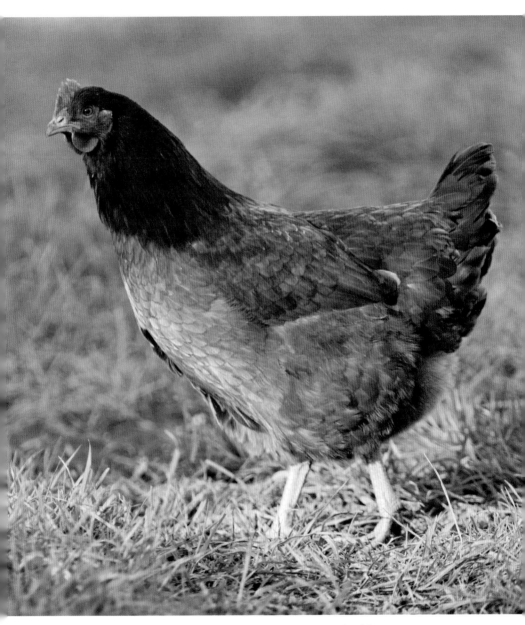

This New Hampshire has the bright pumpkin color popular on New England farms.
A backyard flock of New Hamps will keep a family well supplied with brown eggs.
Dare 2 Dream Farms

DELAWARE

Delawares have white feathers with a sprinkling of barred feathers in the hackle, wings, and tail.

The Delaware is a twentieth-century creation, developed specifically for the growing broiler market in the 1940s and recognized by the APA for exhibition in 1952. Back then, production was as significant as beauty. The Delaware's usefulness was soon eclipsed by the industrial focus on the bottom line, and the Cornish Rock cross replaced it in commercial flocks. Its composite background as a cross-bred bird undermined its popularity in the show ring, and poultry keepers stopped raising it. It all but disappeared.

Fortunately, because it was the result of crossing two Standard breeds, it can be and has been re-created. A few breeders are taking on the challenge and finding eager followers for this vigorous, fast-maturing breed.

Its fine meat, abundant in both flavor and size, recommend it to small poultry production flocks. It's also a respectable layer of pale brown eggs. Delawares are good broody hens and good mothers.

Males are protective and good flock leaders. Although they are brave and free range happily on pasture, they don't fly over the fence and leave home. And the chicks are the cutest ever: tiny fat balls of fluff with a funny, serious look.

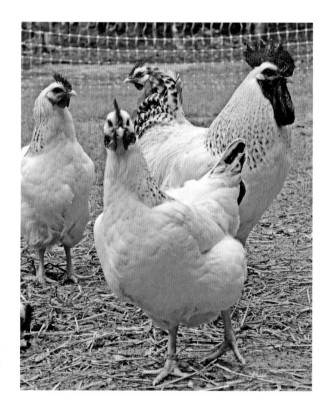

Delawares were developed as commercial meat and egg production birds, but their contrasting black-and-white feathers were so pretty that they were soon welcome in the show ring. Admiring breeders are restoring this American breed to production and show values. *Courtesy of the Livestock Conservancy*

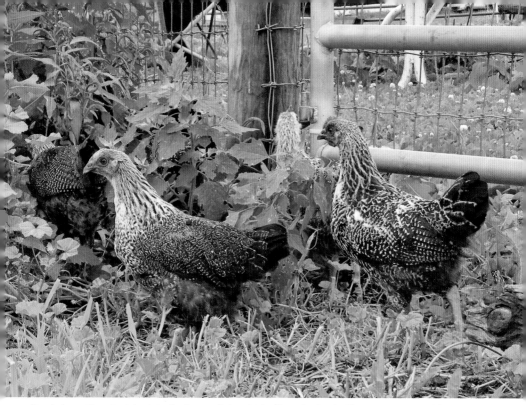

Sturdy Iowa Blues hark back to the farms of the 1920s. They don't mind hot summers or cold winters. They symbolize the innovation and dedication of American farmers to their work.
Kari McKay-Widdel

IOWA BLUE

This flock of chickens looks blue against the green pasture. Looking closer, the hens' feathers are gray with indistinct white and black markings. The rooster is crowned with white feathers down his neck and across his back, setting off his black tail.

History credits a farmer in Decorah, Iowa, with breeding them from Black Minorcas, Rhode Island Reds, and White Plymouth Rocks, with some pheasant thrown in. Pheasants are a separate species and couldn't breed with chickens, but the myth lives on.

Whatever the actual mix, the result is this hardy, beautiful farm breed. They are well adapted to Iowa's harsh weather conditions, hot in the summer and cold in the winter. They are big birds that forage well. They are not intimidated by predators and hunt pests such as mice, rats, and snakes themselves. Their keepers tell tales of roosters defending the flock against hawks and raccoons, and coming out the winner.

These Iowa Blue girls may take note of the first hen who gets broody, and all decide to join her. That brings egg production to a halt, but some breeders consider it one of the strengths of the breed. The hens like raising their own chicks.

They were a popular farm breed from the 1920s to the 1950s, putting eggs and meat on the table, but didn't go to shows. That may change, as the breed has been rediscovered by homesteading families and local food advocates. A breed club is working to achieve APA recognition for Iowa Blues.

PYNCHEON BANTAM

These little charmers won't be confused with any other breed, with a tuft of brilliant light orange vermillion feathers sticking up at the back of the comb, its feathers trailing down its back. It's called a tassel.

Facts about the origins are lost, but Pyncheon bantams date back to the eighteenth century and may have originated in Belgium, where the Mille Fleur color pattern is popular in several breeds. The Pyncheon family name is Flemish.

They claim a literary connection, as Nathaniel Hawthorne writes about them in his novel *House of Seven Gables*. Hawthorne bred them himself, probably when he lived near Lenox, Massachusetts, from 1850 to 1852.

Pyncheons are medium-size bantams, not as tiny as some. Their plumage is the Mille Fleur color pattern. Shanks and toes need to be willow yellow, soles of feet yellow, and earlobes bright red. The Mille Fleur pattern is one of the most difficult to breed to the standard. Like many bantam breeds, they are good layers and good brooders. They lay cream or tinted eggs, are winter hardy, and like to fly.

Pyncheon bantams are recognized by the ABA but not the APA. They are shown in the Single Comb Clean Leg class. Only the bright Mille Fleur variety is recognized, but breeders also raise the porcelain variety: beige and straw yellow with slate blue accents.

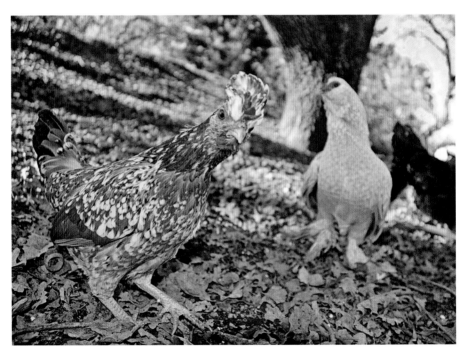

This hearty little Pyncheon hen shows none of the gloomy decline Hawthorne ascribed to the breed. Her plumage is the Mille Fleur color pattern, while the Belgian Bearded d'Uccle hen behind him is the lighter Porcelain color. *Just Struttin' Farm / www.juststruttinfarm.com*

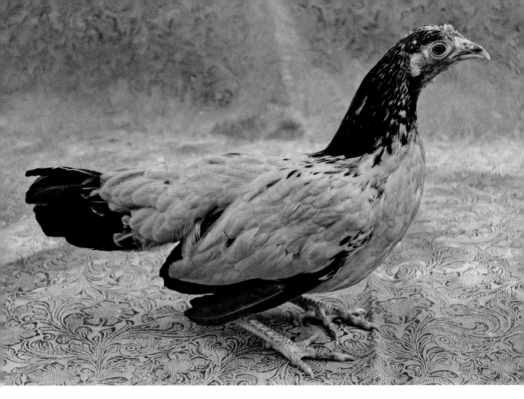

The Vorwerk bantam was developed by a breeder who so admired the large fowl of Germany that he determined to breed a small version in America. It's a rare sighting, but look for the contrasting buff and black feathers. *Courtesy of the Livestock Conservancy*

VORWERK BANTAM

Vorwerks have a unique color pattern featuring buff bodies with black heads, primary wing feathers, and tails. The pattern is so pretty that Wilmar Vorwerk decided he would create them after seeing a picture in a German newspaper back in 1966. None of the large fowl Vorwerks he sought had been imported to the United States, though, so he set about breeding his own. By 1985, the breed was sufficiently perfected to be accepted into the ABA Standard. They are not recognized by the APA.

Vorwerk started by breeding Lakenvelder bantams to Black-Tailed Rosecomb and Buff Wyandotte bantams. The next year he bred a Blue Wyandotte bantam rooster to the first year's pullets. The year after that, he bred selected individuals from the previous year to each other, to improve the color and eliminate rose combs.

Vorwerk added a Buff Columbian Rosecomb bantam rooster to the breeding pen the following year. The offspring had much better color, but about a third of them had rose combs. He continued breeding the best birds to each other until they had the color and comb he wanted and bred true. The effort resulted in a new breed he described as "lively, inquisitive, and beautiful."

Vorwerk bantams are good layers of white eggs, but they find unusual places to lay their eggs. They are the first chicks to find food and water after they hatch. They are curious and active, constantly scratching.

AMERICAN HYBRIDS

Breeders have always crossed breeds to meet their goals: larger size, faster growth, more efficient feed conversion, increased egg production, overcoming weaknesses, and a calm and pleasant disposition.

Hybrids by definition will not reproduce themselves and can look like anything. They can mate and lay and hatch eggs, but the offspring will be mutts, unpredictable in appearance, laying ability, or meat development. One, Rainbow, is sold with the positive spin that no two birds look alike. To have a sustainable flock, traditional breeds are required.

The Cornish/Rock cross is overwhelmingly the chicken hybrid raised for meat. They convert feed into meat faster and at lower cost than any other breed. Cornish crosses are still popular, but not as backyard birds because they do not walk well and are unable to do much except sit by the feed dish and eat. Modern commercial hybrids were developed to produce a chicken that is vigorous enough to forage and enjoy life on pasture. Red Ranger and Silver Cross are other hybrid meat birds.

Egg breeds will continue to lay for several years, although production is highest in the first two or three years. White Leghorns are the most common white egg layer and Rhode Island Reds the most common brown egg layer. Egg hybrids include ISA Browns (Institut de Selection Animale, the company that developed them) and Hy-Line's Brown, Silver Brown, and Sonia.

Many hybrids have registered trademark names, such as Freedom Ranger, Red Ranger, and ISA Browns, or a proprietary name such as Cinnamon Queen, Golden Nugget, or California White. They are commercial products, and that's how they are sold.

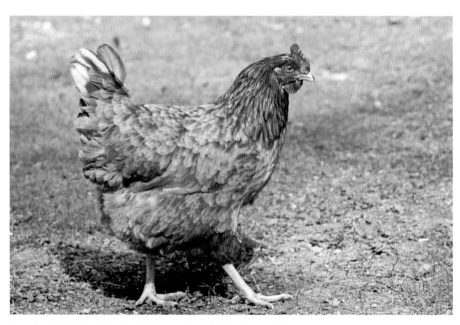

A modern hybrid production chicken such as this Red Star will lay well for several years. They are the result of a red rooster bred to a hen of another breed. Because they are hybrids, they are not show chickens. *Paulette Johnson/Fox Hill Photo*

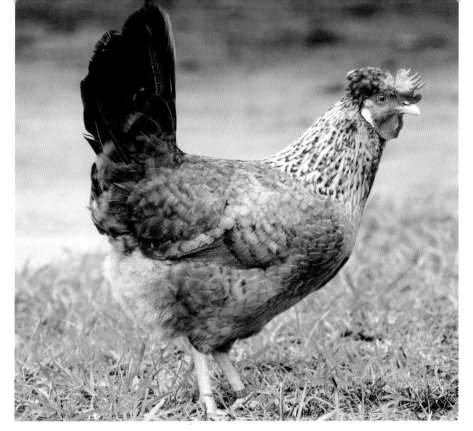

Cream Legbars are a modern twentieth-century English autosexing breed. Note this hen's fluffy crest of feathers behind her red comb. She lays blue, green, or olive eggs, a trait inherited from her Araucana ancestors. *Courtesy Greenfire Farms*

SEX-LINKS

Crossing two breeds of different colors often results in sex-linked chickens. Sex-links are chickens that have distinctively different feather colors on males and females, starting at day one. This provides the advantage of knowing which is which and reducing the chance of acquiring an unwanted rooster. They are the result of crossing different colored parents of Standard breeds. The resulting chicks tend to be hardier and more vigorous than either parent.

Red roosters, such as New Hampshires and Rhode Island Reds, father both red and black sex-links, depending on the mother's color. For black sex-links, a red father on a Barred Rock mother produces black chicks, but males have a white dot on their heads. Females grow up black with a few red feathers, while males grow up looking like Barred Rocks, with a few stray red feathers. They are sometimes called Rock Reds.

Red sex-links result from a red father and a white or mostly white mother, such as White Rock, Silver Laced Wyandotte, Rhode Island White, or Delaware. Female chicks are buff or red and male chicks are white. Popular sex-link hybrids include Golden Comets (New Hampshire on White Rock) and Cinnamon Queen (New Hampshire on Silver Laced Wyandotte).

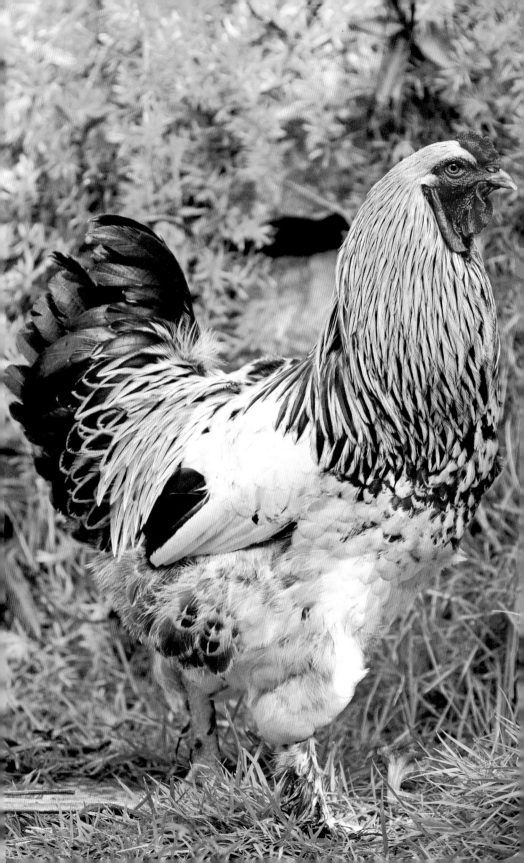

ASIATIC BREEDS

The three Asiatic breeds–Brahma, Cochin, and Langshan–made a sensation when they arrived in the United States in the middle of the nineteenth century. Their size amazed Americans accustomed to smaller and shorter chickens. A. F. Hunter, associate editor of *Reliable Poultry Journal* in the 1920s, remembers Yellow Shanghais, Gray Chittigongs, and Malays from sixty years before, which were "so tall that, while standing on the floor beside it, they could eat corn off the top of a barrel that was standing on end." Those birds may have weighed eighteen pounds. They don't grow them that big any more.

Their unusual colors, especially buff, captured the public eye. Breeders eagerly bred that color into their flocks. Soon buff colored birds of home-grown breeds were being shown. The Asiatic breeds also contributed their soft, fluffy feathers, which now extended down the legs to their feet.

The Asiatics set off the "Hen Fever" craze, when fanciers got so excited and competitive about chickens that they bid each other up, sometimes paying hundreds of dollars for a single bird. Like all bubbles, the inflated price eventually burst and deflated. In 1855, George Pickering Burnham wrote a book about it: *The History of Hen Fever: A Humorous Account.* Burnham also made a lot of money selling birds he raised and was a regular visitor on the New England docks, to get the first pick of new, exciting chickens ship captains brought back from their journeys.

Asiatics are all large, inspiring breeders to breed them into local flocks to get bigger chickens. They lay large brown eggs, some of them in large quantities. Those fine qualities were bred into many other breeds and show their influence in modern breeds.

Hunter recounts the history of the importation of various fowls from Cochin China, a French colony in what is now southern Vietnam. These birds, drawn by Samuel Read, were presented to Queen Victoria in 1843. He refers to Lewis Wright's *New Book of Poultry*, in which Wright refutes the idea that those birds are the antecedents of modern Cochins. They are tall and rangy, more like Malays. They do not have the soft feathers of modern Cochins or feathered feet. Poultry history isn't always well documented, leading to discussion and dispute over which and what came first.

The king of all poultry is the Brahma. This Light Brahma rooster reigns over his backyard flock. His smooth feathers cover a strong body that may weigh twelve pounds. Back in the nineteenth century, his forebears may have weighed eighteen pounds. *Jared Shomo/Shutterstock*

BRAHMA

Brahmas are tall, stately chickens whose brows overshadow their eyes a bit, giving them a serious look. Feathers extend down their legs and cover their feet.

Their fans call them The Majestic Ones. They arrived in New England ports on sailing ships from China in the mid-nineteenth century along with Cochins, followed by Langshans slightly later. Light and Dark Brahmas were included in the first Standard in 1874. The Buff variety was added in 1924.

Light ones are most often seen, with their white bodies topped at neck with black hackle feathers laced with white edges. The body is white, ending with a glossy black tail laced with white accents. This color pattern is known as Columbian in other breeds. Keeping the feathery white feet and legs of Light Brahmas clean takes special effort.

The less frequently encountered Dark Brahma roosters and hens are quite different. The rooster is black from the breast down to the toes, topped with a silvery white back and head, tapering off to black feathers laced with white edges and a lustrous black tail. Each of the hen's feathers is triple-lined with penciled markings, black on steel gray to silvery white.

Black markings on golden feathers differentiate Buff Brahmas. The Buff variety is a later development, created after the buff color became so popular in the late nineteenth century.

Brahmas have a calm disposition and a stately carriage. They are broody and will raise their own chicks and don't mind living indoors if necessary. They need nine months to a year to mature and develop their plumage. Although their large size—twelve pounds for the mature rooster and nine and a half pounds for the mature hen—has made them attractive to flock owners as meat birds, they are also good layers of brown eggs.

The bantam varieties were developed alongside the large fowl in the late nineteenth century. Brahma bantams are large enough to be useful production birds. At thirty-eight ounces for mature males and thirty-four ounces for mature females, they are substantial and make a nice meat bird. Bantams are also popular show birds.

This Light Brahma hen has a stern look, but she is a good mother. Her keeper has kept her white feathers sparkling clean, an achievement especially on her feet. Dare 2 Dream Farms

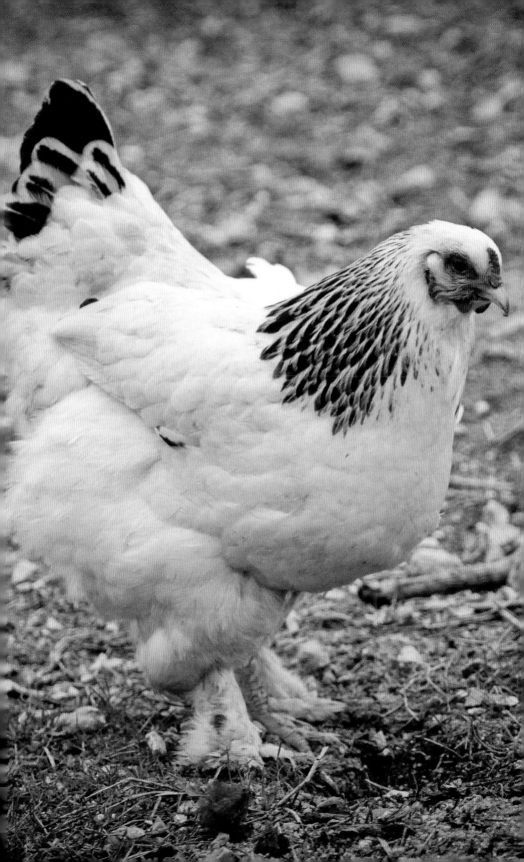

COCHIN

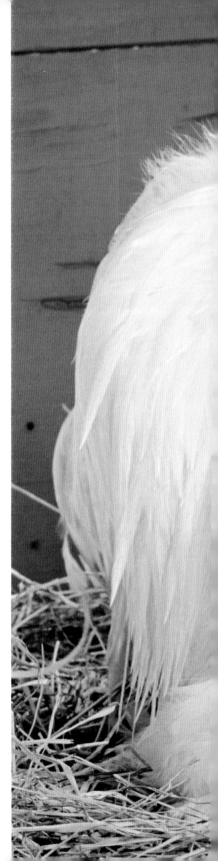

Cochins are big, round puffy chickens, masses of soft feathers creating a rounded silhouette. Their fluffy feathers make them look even larger than they are. The hens are often good broody hens and mothers. Combined with their calm and friendly disposition, they make excellent backyard birds.

A Cochin that looks like it's having a bad hair day may be a frizzle. Frizzled feathers, which curl up and out, can occur in any breed, but breeders are most attracted to them in Cochins, which already have lots of flowing, soft feathers. Some see Cochins as somewhat clownish. Because their feathers completely cover their feet and legs, they look like they are doddering around.

Cochins were developed in the United States from birds imported from, presumably, Shanghai in the nineteenth century. New Englanders, unfamiliar with these new kinds of chickens from China, called them by whatever exotic name suited. The Cochin Craze drove up prices, with some pairs selling for as much as $200.

Cochins are a dual-purpose breed, big for meat and good egg layers. Mostly they are shown as exhibition birds. The American Poultry Association recognizes Buff, Partridge, White, Black, Silver Laced, Golden Laced, Blue, Brown, and Barred varieties of the Cochin. Many unrecognized colors are also raised, including Red, Mottled, and Splash. Seventeen color varieties of bantam Cochins are recognized by the American Bantam Association, including Black Tailed Red, Birchen, Golden Laced, Columbian, Lemon Blue, and Splash. They are second only to the English Game bantam in popularity.

These stylish birds attracted many breeders, and Cochins were bred into many flocks of other breeds, many styles of which were not in the breed's best interest and led to birds with very short legs.

Cochin bantams are the second most popular bantam breed at shows. This white rooster struts his stuff. They are shown in sixteen other feather colors, and devoted breeders raise even more. *Paulette Johnson/Fox Hill Photo*

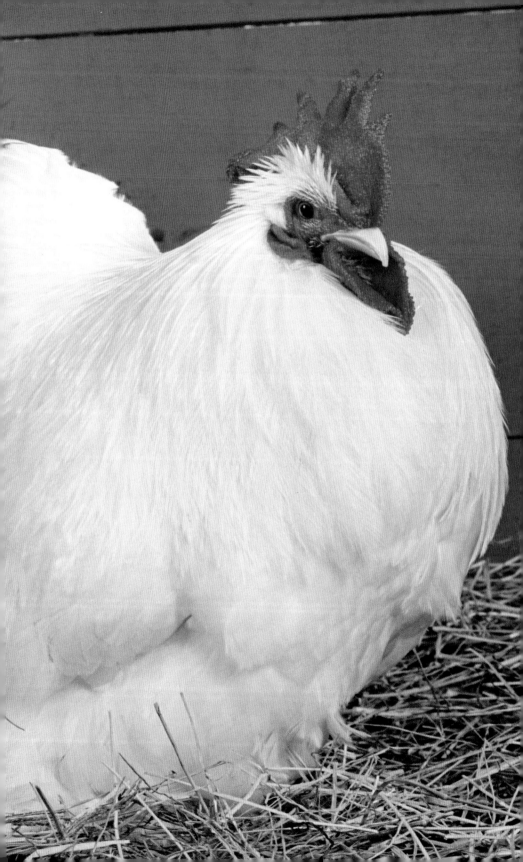

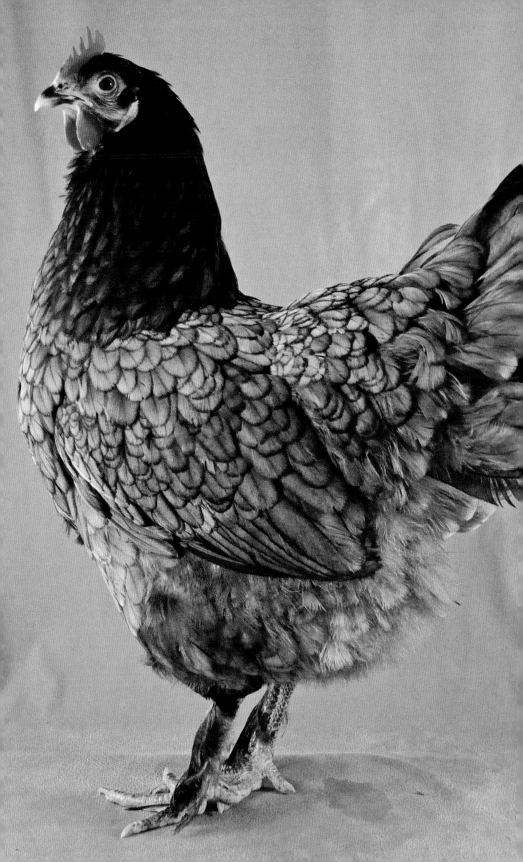

LANGSHAN

Langshans are tall but different from Games. They stand upright, holding their heads high, their silhouette balanced by their flowing tail. Their necks are longer than other breeds. A third of their height comes from the depth of their body. Rooster tail feathers may reach seventeen inches long.

They have feathers down the outer part of their leg all the way to the outer toe, but not the completely feathered-covered feet of the Cochin and less than the Brahma. You may see them in Black, Blue, or White feathers. The black ones glisten iridescent green on the neck, saddle, tail covert, and sickle feathers. The rest of the feathers are black, without the green sheen, but not rusty.

Langshans are gentle around people and other breeds of poultry as well. They are calm and inquisitive and forage well. The hens are good layers of light pinkish brown to dark pinkish brown eggs.

Langshans and Cochins are undoubtedly related, but reached the West from separate geographic areas. Langshans are named for their origin in the five Langshan Hills above Shanghai. The pinnacle hill,

Langshan ("wolf" in Mandarin) Hill is still a nationally prestigious site, known for the Guangjiao Temple, a Buddhist shrine established in the Tang Dynasty, and the view overlooking the Yangtse River from its southern bank.

The Langshan breed was first brought to England in 1872 by Major Croad from China. In England, Croad Langshans are still specified as a variety in the English Standard. E. A. Samuels, an ornithologist, of Waltham, Massachusetts, brought them to the United States in 1876. I. K. Felch wrote the original Langshan standard and worked to get the breed recognized in 1883.

When Langshans first arrived in the United States, their wings were big enough to let them fly. Today, their wings are medium size, but some Langshan hens have wings large enough that they can and do fly. Roosters do not fly, but it's not clear whether flying is aerodynamically impossible for them or temperamentally disdained.

Langshans are rarely kept now, but are an admirable breed for show, utility, or a beautiful backyard flock.

This Blue Langshan hen stands tall but has a fluid grace. Her feathers have dark outlines called lacing. Note that feathers grow down the outer sides of her legs. Courtesy of the Livestock Conservancy

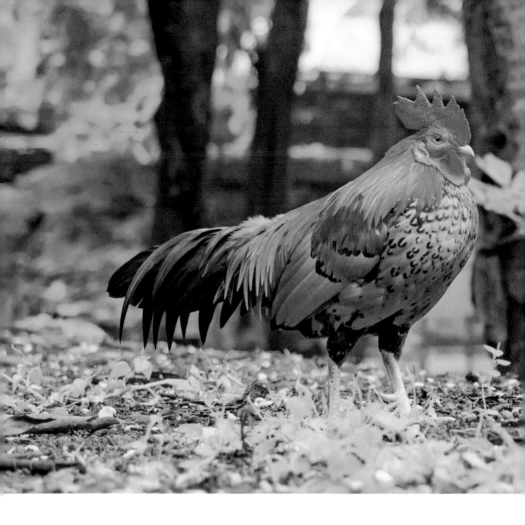

JUNGLEFOWL

Approach Junglefowl cautiously, or they will flap away in alarm. They retain a whiff of the wildness of their ancestral home in Indian and Southeast Asian jungles. They are small, with the roosters brightly colored and the females camouflaged by plumage to disguise them while nesting on the ground.

Topped by a reddish orange head on blazing red-orange neck feathers that flash gold at the edges, Red Junglefowl cocks overshadow their plain hens. Their black breasts glisten in contrast with their red

backs. Hens are drab, as are other ground-nesting female birds. Their single, upright serrated combs are small; their wattles and earlobes are barely noticeable.

Junglefowl are recognized by the ABA but not the APA for exhibition. Captive birds are raised and shown. In captivity, Junglefowl naturally grow larger than they do in the wild. That small size is important for show flocks.

If you encounter Junglefowl in the summer, you may not be able to tell the males from the females. It's called an

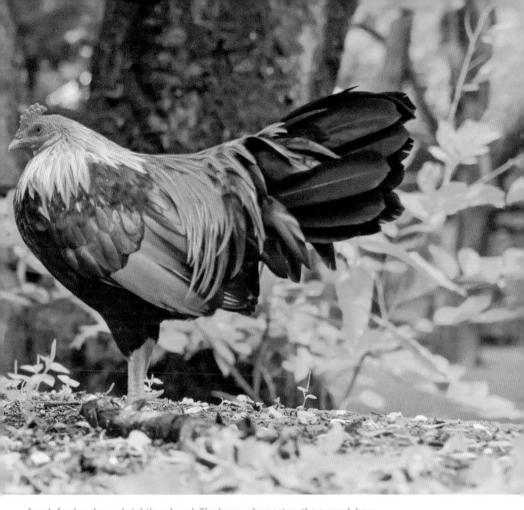

Junglefowl cocks are brightly colored. The hens, who nest on the ground, have drab plumage that camouflages them. In the wild, Junglefowl are smaller than these boys. Junglefowl tend to grow larger in captivity. *Nopparatz/Shutterstock*

eclipse molt, when the male molts to the drab appearance of the hen.

Their plumage isn't standardized the way other domesticated breeds are. Only the Red species is kept and shown. Variations among regional varieties, or subspecies, are sufficient to have separate names: Cochin-Chinese, Burmese, Tonkinese, and Javan. They have dark, usually slate, legs.

Junglefowl's four species—Ceylon Junglefowl, Gray Junglefowl, Java or Green Junglefowl, and Red—interbreed, but with varying degrees of fertility. Many still live in the wild in India, although crossing with domestic poultry threatens their genetic purity. The geography of Asia keeps the various species separate. The Red Junglefowl is the primary ancestor of modern domestic chickens, and DNA has been identified in bones of domesticated chickens dated more than ten thousand years ago in China.

They all are social and live in flocks, but with variations in social structure. Some form mated pairs for life and some males maintain harems. Red Junglefowl roosters naturally prefer to protect a flock of several hens.

SILKIE

Silkies' hair-like feathers are unique and differentiate them from all other chicken breeds. The feathers do not have the barbicels, or little hooks, which make feathers connect in a web. Those hair-like feathers require special care. They don't resist water the way other chicken feathers do. Silkies can get soaked through, get chilled, and die. They have to stay out of the rain.

Their heads are downy-soft fluffy balls, with feathers mushrooming up into a puffball. They have feathered crests on their heads. Bearded varieties have feathers from their eyes down to their throats but non-bearded varieties don't. A beard is the cluster of feathers on the throat, under the beak. Muffs are the feathers on the sides, all joined together from the eyes down to the throat.

Their earlobes are turquoise blue. Their face, walnut comb, and wattles are dark purple, around a blue beak. Less obvious is their black or dark violet skin and, underneath it all, black meat and bones. They have five toes, where most chickens have only four, covered in feathers.

Silkies are probably the breed described by Marco Polo from his experiences in China between 1276 and 1291, where he saw " . . . a kind of fowls which have no feathers, but hair only, like a cat's fur." The only ones he saw were black.

Silkies are small and shown in bantam classes at APA shows and in ABA shows. The original color included in the 1874 Standard, White in both bearded and non-bearded varieties, remains the most popular. The White is the pure heritage Silkie. Six additional colors, in bearded and non-bearded varieties, are recognized.

Aside from their unusual appearance, they are known for their endearing disposition. They are generally calm and friendly and make good pets. Traditional Chinese healers value them for the therapeutic benefits of black chicken meat for soup and other medicinal uses.

Hens are often broody, sometimes annoyingly so, and even roosters will care for chicks. Breeders often keep a few Silkie hens to hatch eggs when their non-sitters won't. When they do lay, their eggs are small and either white or light brown.

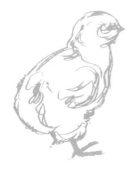

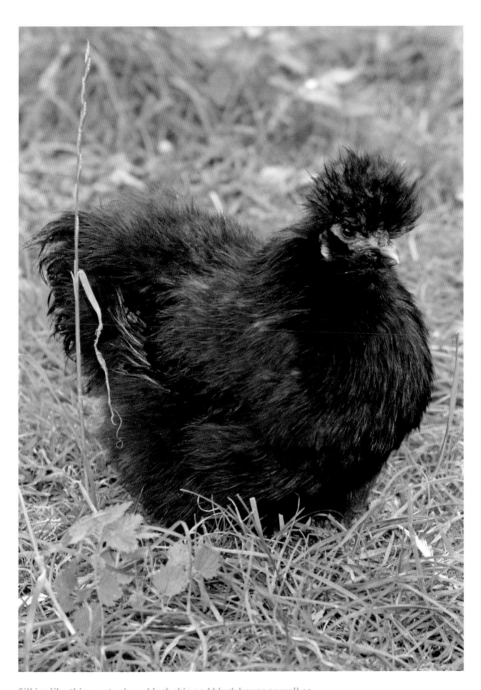

Silkies like this rooster have black skin and black bones as well as black, hair-like feathers. He has a beard and muffs—the feathers around his face and under his beak. You can see why they are one of the most popular bantams. *Erni/Shutterstock*

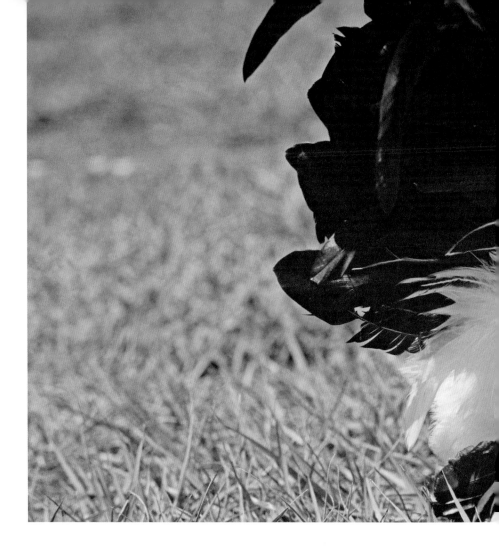

JAPANESE BANTAM

Japanese bantams are tiny birds that toddle around on their short legs and are so small that their wings can easily carry them up into the trees. Folded, their wings sweep down gracefully, nearly touching the ground. Their tails tower over their backs, nearly touching their heads. Their bright red combs, although large for small birds, balance that magnificent tail. The flock shows off many colors, but most have black tails that contrast with buff or white bodies. Some are all white, and some are all black.

Japanese bantams are delicate, requiring protection from the elements and a warm coop in the winter. Wet weather and a muddy run can damage their feathers. They need clean bedding and dry roosts, not too far off the ground, to keep their feathers in show condition. Otherwise, they are friendly, easy to care for, and make good pets. The hens lay plenty of tiny brown eggs. They are good broody hens and attentive mothers.

Japanese bantams are a true bantam, with no large fowl correlate. Because of

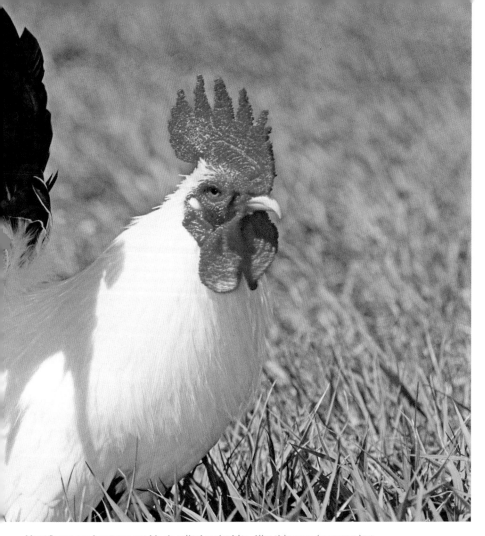

Most Japanese bantams are black-tailed and white, like this proud rooster, but breeders raise them in more than a dozen other colors. Their unusually high tail and short legs make them special. *Paulette Johnson/Fox Hill Photo*

the genetic allele combination for short legs, breeding can be a challenge, and breeding a short-legged female to a short-legged male results in about a quarter of the chicks dead in the shell before they hatch. Half of the eggs in the clutch will hatch short-legged birds. The remaining quarter will have long legs, disqualifying them from the show ring. Breeding the shortest to those with longer legs prevents inbreeding faults and infertility.

In other breeds, that tail might be considered a squirrel tail, a disqualification.

Not so for Japanese bantams. Their fourteen main tail feathers are topped by long sickle feathers, curved like a Japanese sword. They have a long history in Japan, arriving there from Vietnam, Thailand, and Malaysia in the early seventeenth century. The ABA recognizes seventeen color varieties, including a White Bearded variety. The APA recognizes nine. The Black-Tailed White, still the most popular was included in the first Standard of Excellence in 1874.

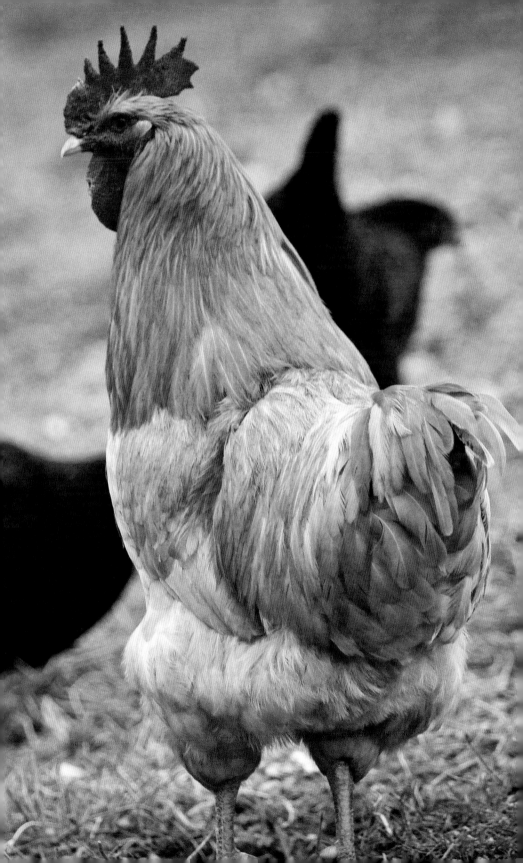

ENGLISH BREEDS

English chicken breeds have glorified barnyards for centuries. Chickens were being kept by Romans occupying England two thousand years ago, but the Celts who already inhabited the British Isles probably had their own chickens, most likely Game types.

The British Poultry Standards continue a proud history of maintaining beauty and economic value for many poultry breeds. In the United States, six breeds are so closely identified with Britain that they have their own English class: Dorkings, Redcaps, Cornish, Orpingtons, Sussex, and Australorps. Two true bantams are also English: Rosecombs and Sebrights.

English settlers brought their birds with them to America as colonists as far back as the sixteenth century. Those birds were part of the colonial scene, feeding their keepers with meat and eggs, growing up scraping away at the dung hill and keeping bugs under control in the barnyard. As the exhibition fancy took hold in the nineteenth century, chickens were traded back and forth across the Atlantic, sharing traits developed on one side with the other.

All English breeds except the Cornish have white skin. This has become cultural—even the grocery store chickens in England are white rather than yellow. Like the color of egg shells, it makes no difference in flavor or nutrition. It's purely cosmetic for the consumer.

This Buff Orpington is the most popular color of the Orpington breed. Orpingtons are popular in Black, White, and Blue plumage too. *Dare 2 Dream Farms*

DORKING

Dorkings are the classic breed, historically the Five-Toed Fowl of England, the meat bird of the English-speaking world. They take their name from the English market town of Dorking in Surrey, which now has a museum in their honor. But historic evidence shows that the breed predates English farms.

Dorkings may have been introduced to England by the Romans, as the breed is clearly depicted in Roman mosaics and described by Roman writers of the first century AD. Other historians set the date of their arrival in England later, to 1066 with the Norman conquest. A breed with such a long history is inevitably of historical interest and discussion. Not limited to the United Kingdom and United States, Dorking fanciers have breed clubs in Australia and New Zealand as well as Europe and North America. Dorking-like fowl have been found in Southern China and Bangladesh.

Three colors were originally recognized in 1874: Colored, Silver-Gray, and White. Although the Red variety was not recognized in the Standard until 1995, it's considered the color variety with the longest history. Cuckoo Dorkings, with black and white barred feathers like Dominiques, another old breed, achieved APA recognition in both single and rose comb varieties in 2001. It is one of the few breeds for which both single and rose comb varieties are recognized for exhibition. Other color varieties include Dark Birchen Gray, Brown Red, Light Gray, Spangled, Clay, Dark Red, and Black.

Dorkings are still dual-purpose birds, hefty as meat birds at nine pounds for a mature rooster and seven pounds for a mature hen. They lay well, with eggs that are porcelain or lightly tinted rather than chalk white. Dorkings are one of the exceptions to the rule that chickens with red earlobes lay brown eggs.

They take six to seven months to come to market size, producing a three-and-a-half to four-and-a-half-pound carcass.

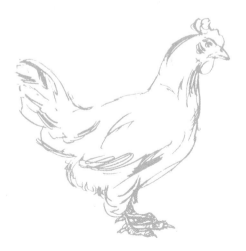

Note this Dorking rooster's fifth toe, growing out of the back of his white leg. It's a distinctive trait, as most chickens have only four toes.
marilyn barbone/Shutterstock

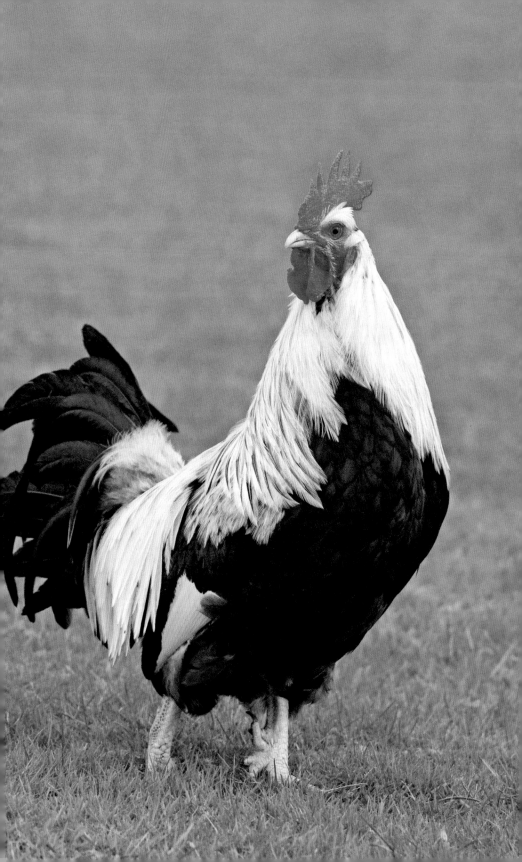

CORNISH

That blocky fellow, so muscle-bound he rocks from side to side as he walks, legs planted wide apart—that's a Cornish.

Their heads are strong, with a small pea comb and small wattles. They hold their short, hard feathers close, bringing out their vibrant colors and showing off their muscular physique. Dark Cornish glisten iridescent green on their black feathers, with accents of red. The hen shines mahogany red, with those greenish black edges to her feathers. Pure White, Buff, and White Laced Red varieties are also recognized by the APA. Cornish bantams are one of the ABA's ten most popular breeds, shown in a dozen recognized colors. Cornish are one of the largest bantam chickens, at nearly three pounds for roosters and over two pounds for hens.

They are inclined to gain weight—the meat producer's goal—but that is not any healthier for chickens than it is for people. Their natural inclination to develop muscle can also put on fat, which interferes with fertility and egg production. See them active on pasture, where they can eat plenty of grass to keep their legs and feet bright yellow.

Taller roosters may be bred to the ideal short-legged hens, to keep the flock vigorous.

The Cornish takes its name from Cornwall in England, on the southwest coast. Originally, they were Indian Games, descended from Aseels and Malays. The breed was recognized in England in 1886, and at least a trio were bought to the United States in 1877. The APA recognized them as Cornish in 1893.

Cornish-Rock crosses, the most popular industrial hybrid, are not good backyard chickens. They are highly bred for low food conversion ratio, which means they gain more weight on less feed than other breeds and are ready for slaughter at six to seven weeks old. They are not suited to life on pasture and often suffer from leg and other skeletal problems, cardiac diseases, and immune deficiency that makes them susceptible to disease.

The industrial Cornish-Rock cross is the most influential bird in American poultry. The Cornish-Rock cross is the chicken found in every grocery store. They are far from the traditional standard Cornish. The standard Cornish is a vibrant, healthy, beautiful chicken that would make any backyard flock owner proud.

This Dark Cornish hen shows her heritage as a stocky meat breed. Heritage breed Cornish influenced the industrial meat birds today. In England, Cornish were originally known as Indian Games. *Paulette Johnson/Fox Hill Photo*

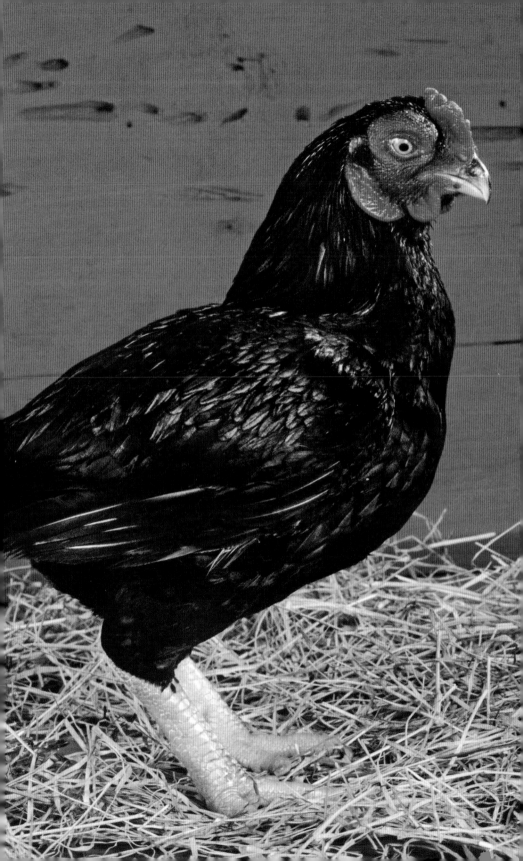

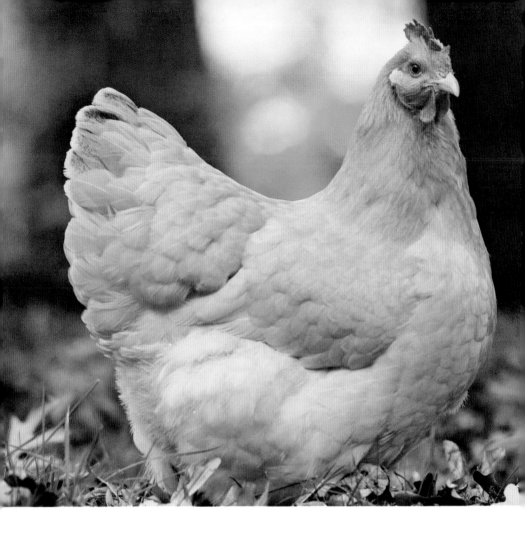

ORPINGTON

An Orpington's silhouette shows a U-shaped back and a perfectly straight comb with five spikes. They're big, but not so massive as the Cornish.

The name comes from the town Orpington in the County of Kent, England, where this breed was developed in the late nineteenth century. This breed is credited to William Cook, who was dissatisfied with the quality of the old breeds around him. He wanted to create a breed that would lay well, be large enough and tasty for the table, and beautiful enough to show.

Mr. Cook selected black sports from Barred Rock matings that often laid more eggs than their barred parents as the basis for his new breed. He bred those black Plymouth Rocks to Black Minorcas, then their daughters to Black Langshan roosters. As he crossed roosters of one breed with hens of another, he observed that their offspring laid more eggs than their purebred parents.

It took years to refine the Orpington into a distinct breed, losing those Langshan leg feathers and settling on a single comb. The breed was welcomed to the poultry world, spreading around the world within twenty years after the original black was introduced in 1886.

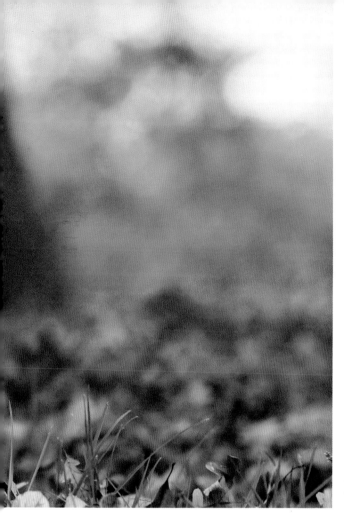

Orpingtons are a distinguished English breed. The buff color is best known, but they may be black, white, or blue. Orpingtons have been a favorite of the English royal family for generations. *Amy Kerkemeyer/Shutterstock*

White Orpingtons followed, developed from white Leghorn roosters and black Hamburg hens. Their daughters were mated to a single-comb white Dorking.

Blue Orpingtons result from breeding black to white Orpingtons. One quarter of the offspring will be black, one-quarter splash, and half of them will be the intended blue. It's a numbers game.

To develop the buff variety, Mr. Cook mated a Golden-Spangled Hamburg cock to Dark Dorking pullets. Their daughters were bred to a buff Cochin rooster. It took ten years to refine to the Orpington body shape and consistent color. Buff

Orpingtons may have looser feathers even today, reflecting their Cochin heritage. In the United States, the APA recognized the Buff variety in 1902, the Black and the White in 1905, and the Blue in 1923.

Orpingtons come in many other colors that are not yet recognized. In England, colors raised include Gold Laced, Cuckoo, Lemon Cuckoo, Lavender, Porcelain, and Splash. Recently, Chocolate Orpingtons have attracted attention in Internet sales, but reports have varied, so buyer beware.

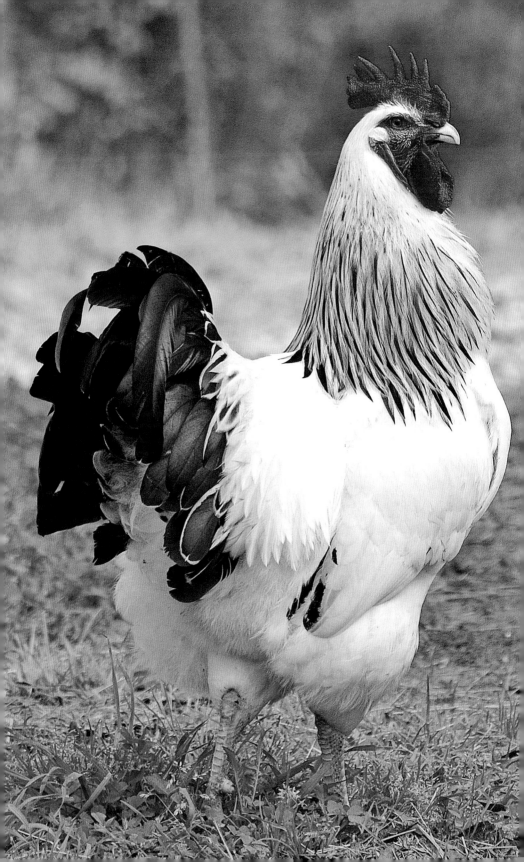

SUSSEX

Any speckled chicken you see is probably a Sussex. White and black speckles on each rich dark red mahogany bay feather gives the Speckled Sussex unusual, eye-catching plumage. They have that white English skin, and hold their tails at a 45-degree angle, giving them a sprightly look. They are hardy and resourceful, eager foragers that stay healthy and lay brown eggs well. They don't mind the cold and are good setters and mothers.

As an old barnyard breed, Sussex come in other colors, some of which are recognized for showing in the United States: Red and Light for large fowl; Birchen, Buff, Dark Brown, and White for bantams. Others are recognized in England, such as Coronation, White, and Buff. Coronation Sussex, in which the black accents in the neck and tail of the Light variety are replaced with silvery lavender, was developed to honor the coronation of Edward VIII. That heralded event did not come to be, because he abdicated the throne to marry Wallis Simpson in 1936.

Sussex are named for an English county, harking back to the days when farmers bred birds with distinctive plumage to make them easy to identify if they were stolen. Cock fighting influenced the development of breeds, as tenant farmers were allowed to keep chicks fathered by the landowner's fighting cocks, so long as none of them had a Game hen for a mother. Tenant farmers kept the young roosters with their flocks of local hens, keeping all the Game/barnyard cross chickens that resulted.

Kent, Surrey, and Dorking chickens are similar, all also taking their names from English locations where farmers took pride in their chickens. As breeds became standardized for show classifications in the mid-nineteenth century, Sussex were bred to a distinctive character. The popular Brahmas and Cochins of that time arrived from China at Sussex seaports, and farmers welcomed them into their flocks, adding size to what had been a smaller barnyard fowl. Light Brahmas especially can be seen in Light Sussex, which tend to be larger and fluffier than other Sussex varieties.

Although they were not admitted to the APA Standard until 1914 (Red and Speckled) and the Light variety in 1929, their history is long and honorable.

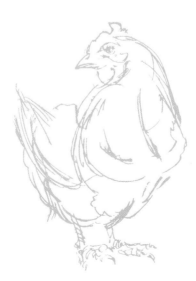

The Sussex represents a long history of chicken breeding. This color pattern, called Light, is called Columbian in other breeds—the only difference is that his back is solid white.
Courtesy Greenfire Farms

AUSTRALORP

Australorps are big, black chickens that are slightly smaller than Orpington, Jersey Giants, and Javas. They're Australia's version of an egg-producing Orpington. While Orpingtons were being bred as meat breeds in England in the late nineteenth and early twentieth centuries, Australians were competing for egg production. The Orpingtons imported Down Under were soon known as Australian Utility Orpingtons. That name got shortened to Australs and eventually Australorp was the accepted name. They were recognized as a breed by the APA in 1929.

The original Orpingtons had harder feathers, like today's Australorp. One early developer added Black Cochins to his flock, and the showier birds that resulted took the spotlight at English poultry shows. They laid fewer eggs, but winning those prizes trumped that. The egg-producing utility line became the Australorps.

The Australorp triumphed in the egg laying trial conducted at Bendigo, near Melbourne, Australia, in the early 1920s. The record was set by a hen who laid 339 eggs in 365 days. Their eggs are tinted, lighter than the brown to dark brown eggs of Orpingtons, Jersey Giants, and Javas.

Australorps are hardy, attractive, and adaptable to climate, although they lay less in colder climes. Australorps lost ground to more exotic heritage breeds but are an excellent utility chicken happy in small backyard flocks.

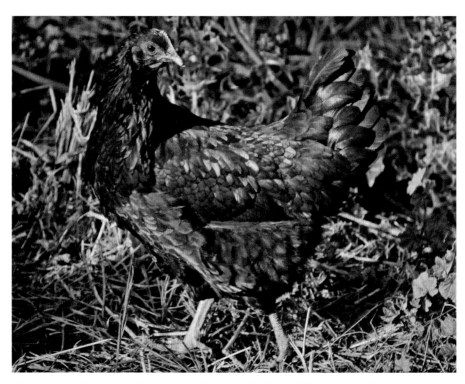

This Australorp is the Australian version of England's Orpington. Watch as Australorps work the yard for their food. They keep busy eating worms and kitchen waste and laying lots of tinted eggs. *Dare 2 Dream Farms*

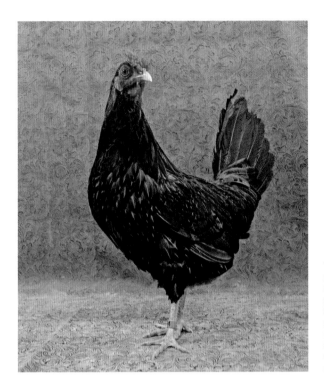

This Redcap hen has an attractive comb, but Redcap roosters have, as their name suggests, a huge comb. English farmers of centuries past valued them for their eggs, but those combs were surely bragging points as well. *Courtesy of the Livestock Conservancy*

REDCAP

This chicken is the crowned king (and queen) of poultry. A prize Redcap rooster's comb back in the nineteenth century measured more than five inches long by more than three inches wide, a hen's nearly three inches by two inches.

That fancy red comb should be symmetrical, with many points and a spike at the back. The hen's is the same as the rooster's but smaller. Although the comb is large, it should be proportional to the size of the entire bird.

Those big combs have distinguished Redcaps through their long history in England, but their path isn't well documented. They are related to Hamburgs, although today's Redcaps are larger. Perhaps it goes the other way, that the Redcap is the original Golden-Spangled Hamburg. They have also been called mongrel Dorkings. The Dorking's

fifth toe occasionally shows up in Redcap flocks. Others think the Redcap resulted from crossing Hamburgs with Old English Games. All those breeds, before they even had their formal names, were common on English farms, so perhaps some of all contributed to this breed.

Roosters are black with red accents. Hens have brown on their backs and spangled feathers. They are hardy, good foragers, active, and alert. Redcaps are an exception to the general rule that chickens with red earlobes lay brown eggs. They have red earlobes, with a white dot in the center, but lay white eggs. Their fame was for their eggs, not only quantity but size and quality. They are large birds also popular for the table, more a classic dual-purpose farm chicken than the small egg producing Hamburg.

ROSECOMB BANTAM

A tiny chicken with large white earlobes, a nice spike at the back of its rose comb, and a wide-spread tail is a Rosecomb bantam. The APA recognized them in 1874 and only accepts three varieties (Black, Blue, and White); the ABA recognizes twenty-six.

This is an exhibition breed. They don't lay many eggs, the hens aren't willing to set and hatch them, and they are too small to be meat birds for the table. For the dedicated fancier, this is a highly refined breed that brings rewards at the most demanding levels of poultry shows.

Because they're one of the top ten most popular bantams, competition for the best Rosecomb at poultry shows is stiff. Breeders often mate the best roosters to both the best-colored hens and to plain hens with dull color. The male offspring of the dull females are often the best colored, while the best colored females are daughters of the brightly colored hens.

They are small and have large wings, so they fly well. Roosters can be aggressive toward each other, to the extent of injuring each other, which can mar a bird otherwise destined for the show ring. Away from the show, you may see Rosecombs kept separate from each other to avoid any detraction from top show condition. A small flock with a single rooster can be happily kept in a backyard.

Rosecombs were already long established, probably dating back before 1450, when they caught the attention of King Richard III in 1483 at the Angel Inn in Grantham, Lincolnshire. His royal attention made them a popular breed even then.

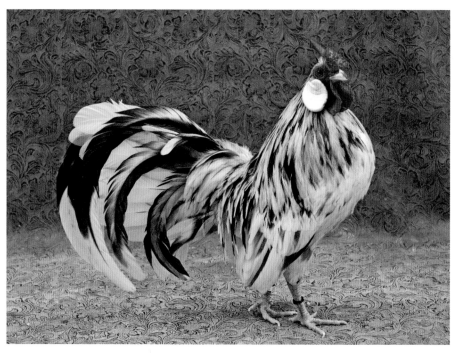

Many chickens have rose combs, but the Rosecomb bantam breed is named for it. Note this rooster's perfectly formed comb, with rounded points over the base and a clean spike in back. You may see them in twenty-six color varieties. *Courtesy of the Livestock Conservancy*

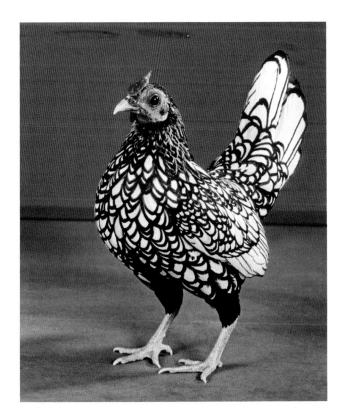

Sebrights are a true bantam—a breed that exists only in its small size—only a pound and a quarter for this little hen. Her distinctive markings make her one of the ten most popular bantam show breeds. *Paulette Johnson/Fox Hill Photo*

SEBRIGHT BANTAM

Tiny chickens with feathers, either golden or pure white, so carefully outlined in black as to look as if an artist had painted them, are Sebrights. Their short backs and tails held high give them a sporty look. Males and females have the same color feathers, called henny feathering. Their purplish-red facial skin sets off their dark brown eyes, under a purplish-red rose comb ending in a nice spike. Earlobes may share the purplish-red of the face or be turquoise.

Sebrights are an exhibition breed, laying only small eggs and being too small for meat. Fertility is low, which may be genetically related to the rose comb or may be due to inbreeding. Occasional single-combed sports, disqualified for showing, may be included in breeding to improve fertility.

They are named for Sir John Sebright, who developed them around 1800 in London. He started with a small buff bantam hen (perhaps a Nankin), a reddish henny Game cockerel, and a small Golden Hamburg type hen. Sebright added a White Rosecomb cockerel he got from the London Zoo. Black Rosecombs may have also gone into the mix, to keep the birds small. By 1812, Sebrights and their unusual markings were capturing the interest of other English breeders.

They were included in the APA's first Standard of Perfection in 1874, already a popular breed.

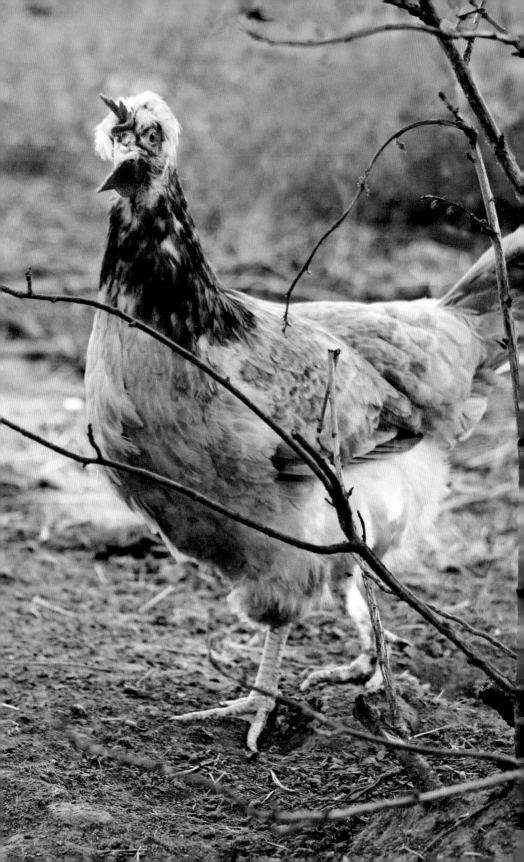

CRESTED BREEDS

The fluffy fountain of feathers tumbling over crested chickens' faces has attracted plenty of attention over the years. The crest is sometimes called a topknot or a top hat. That knob isn't just feathers up there. Crested breeds have a dome of bone on their skulls. The feathers grow out of that. Because of the placement of the crest, the bony skull structure affects the nostrils, so that crested chickens have flattened, cavernous nostrils.

The small Polish is the most popular breed of crested chicken. Crèvecoeurs are larger, always all black, and show a distinctive horned comb with two prongs. Houdans are usually mottled black and white and have a fifth toe, a spur on the back of the leg. Hefty Sulmtaler roosters have a small tuft at the back of the serrated comb, but hens have a nice crest and their combs meander in an *S* shape on their heads. Brabanters and Appenzeller Spitzhaubens have pointy crests behind that V comb. Sultans are petite white chickens with feathers down their legs as well as all over their heads.

Although their appearance invites humor, crested chickens have a long and distinguished history and are honored for their productive usefulness as well.

Crests require extra care. Breeders may trim the crest back or hold it back with a rubber band during breeding season so the birds can see what they are doing. Special waterers can help the bird avoid getting the crest and beard feathers soaked, which can ruin them for a show.

The crested breeds have *V* combs, even if they are concealed beneath the crest feathers. The *V* or horn comb, required for exhibition in the United States, is unusual. In England and France, the leaf comb, shaped like butterfly wings, is still recognized. Leaf combs are the result of the *V* comb crossed with a single comb.

This Sulmtaler's crest surrounds the unusual *S*-shaped "wickel" comb. Sulmtalers originated in the Styrian wine country of Austria, taking their name from the Sulm Valley. Their meat and eggs graced royal tables in past centuries.
Brigitte Riemer/Getty Images

POLISH

These chickens aren't necessarily from Poland, although some undoubtedly were raised there. Italian Aldrovandi called them Paduan, which could have referred to the city of Padua. The name may also have referred to that knob, as in polled cattle. Or it could have come from the custom of pollarding trees, the poll being the round knob that grows after branches are pruned back.

The crest is the distinguishing feature. It's full and round. Polish may have no comb at all, or only a small one covered by the crest feathers.

Polish chickens were popular through the centuries as good layers of white eggs. Four varieties were included in the first Standard in 1874, with four more following in 1883. The others are more recent additions. Today, Polish chickens are raised in seven color varieties, both bearded and non-bearded. A beard is the cluster of feathers on the throat, under the beak. Muffs are the feathers on the sides, joining the beard to cover the face from the eyes down to the throat.

The frizzle gene can be bred into any breed, making the feathers curve and curl. Frizzles are shown as a separate class but are judged according the breed standards. Polish chickens tempt breeders to breed that frizzle gene into them.

Polish have their own subclass within the Continental class. Feather color may be uniform all over the bird, such as Golden, Silver, White, and Buff Laced, or may be different on the crest and the rest of the bird, such as White Crested Black and White Crested Blue. Bantams are also recognized in Blue, White Crested Cuckoo, and White Crested Chocolate.

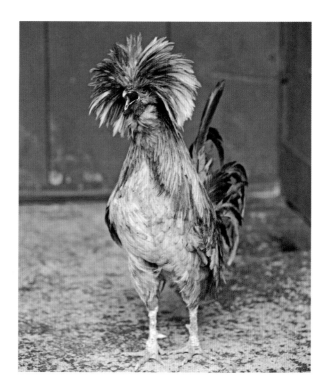

Polish chickens, with their feathery crests, look crazy but are no more excitable than other chickens. That crest can be the same color as the rest of the plumage or a contrasting color, such as white on a black chicken. *MISHELLA/Shutterstock*

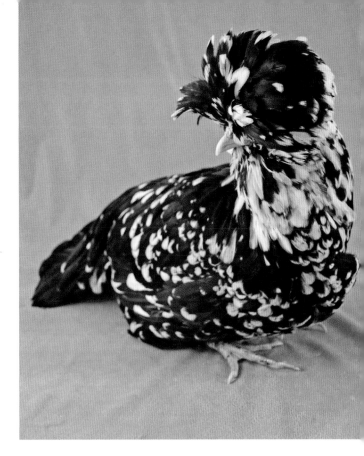

Note the subtle differences between the Crèvecoeur's crest and crests of other breeds, such as the Polish and the Houdan. Crèvecoeurs are always black. Crèvecoeurs were popular in France in the nineteenth century but are now a rare backyard sighting. *Courtesy of the Livestock Conservancy*

CRÈVECOEUR

Crèvecoeurs were developed in France as dual-purpose fowl and were included in the original 1874 APA Standard, though the breed's history dates back to the seventeenth century. The Crèvecoeur is a large bird, topping out at eight pounds for roosters and seven pounds for hens. Both large fowl and bantams are recognized by the APA for exhibition, and bantams by the ABA. As large fowl, they're in the same weight standard as Houdans, but among bantams, Crèvecoeurs are smaller than Houdans, about the same size as Polish.

The Crèvecoeur has a crest and a V comb, although earlier in history they also had leaf combs. The crest feathers incline backward, behind that horned comb. Currently recognized only in black plumage, white and blue were raised in the past. The Crèvecoeur also served as a production fowl in the late nineteenth and early twentieth centuries. They were known for their white bones and meat and lay white eggs. They were so popular that at the Universal Exhibition in Paris in 1855, only two prizes were awarded for poultry: one for the Crèvecoeur and the other for all other breeds of poultry.

HOUDAN

Houdans have also been known as Normandy fowl and were developed from early French market chickens. Historically, they were considered one of the best table fowl breeds as well as good egg layers.

Houdans are recognized in the original mottled black-and-white and the newer (1914) solid white varieties. Mottled birds have black feathers, about a third to a half with *V*-shaped white tips. Their crests are black and white. Solid black, blue mottled, and red mottled varieties have existed in the past and may still be raised by fanciers. Houdan origins may include both Polish and Dorkings, popular breeds in seventeenth-century France. They are sometimes called the Dorkings of France, for their short legs, light bones, and that fifth toe. They share the *V* comb with Crèvecoeurs and Sultans.

Polish are often used as a cross to increase Houdan crests, but Polish crosses will be smaller. White Houdans were developed by crossing the mottled ones with White Polish and White Dorkings. They are now recognized as both large fowl and bantams, but few raise them.

Good Houdans should be hefty birds, at eight pounds for a rooster and six and a half pounds for a hen. Crèvecoeurs have been used to add black feathering to Houdans, which may become almost completely white with age, but white Houdans are rare.

With both beards and muffs, the feathered faces of Houdans require some extra care. The birds need easy access to fresh water without getting their feathers wet. If they get dirty, they should be washed and dried so that they don't interfere with the bird's ability to eat and drink.

Mottled Houdans, with black and white feathering like this one, are the most likely sighting. American Houdans have *V*-shaped combs hidden by the crest, but European ones may have elaborate butterfly combs. *Courtesy of the Livestock Conservancy*

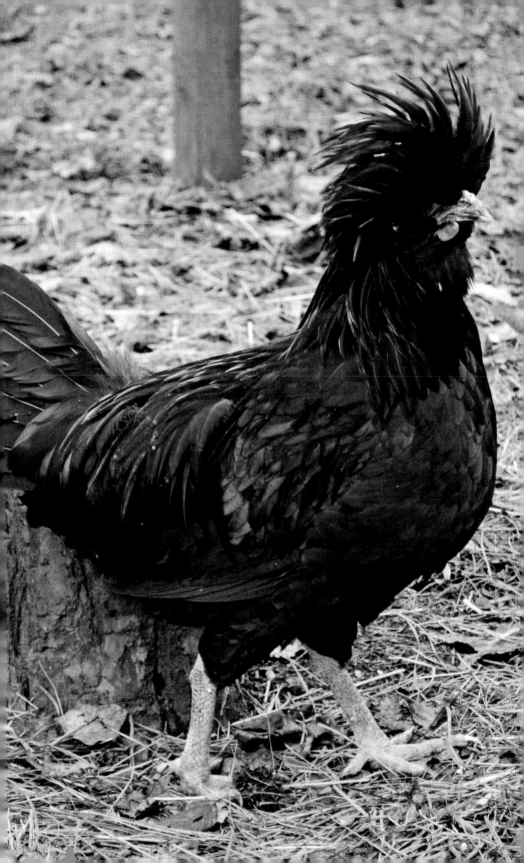

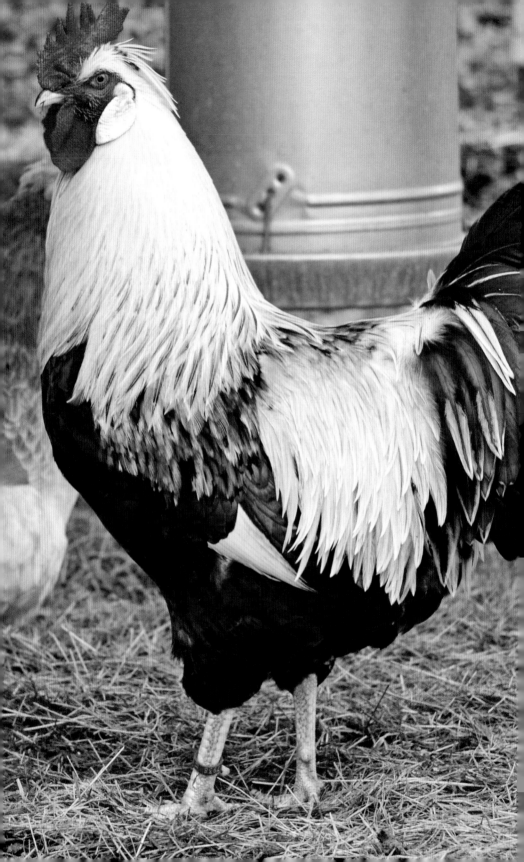

SULMTALER

Sulmtalers take their place-name from the River Sulm in southeastern Austria. They are substantial birds, plump and often corn-fed for a delicious roast chicken or an even larger capon. So good, Sulmtalers were the gourmet choice for French and Austrian nobility in the nineteenth century.

They got their size from local birds bred with Cochins, Houdans, and Dorkings, which also contributed their short legs. The traditional Wheaten color pattern gives roosters bright metallic colors and gold hackles flowing over a rich red back, with a black breast below. Dainty hens are creamy, with orange necks and brown wings.

The depredation of war took its toll on this breed in the twentieth century, but dedicated breeders rescued it. University breeding programs found pure lines that had survived two world wars in the remote Stiermarken region.

As beautiful as they are, they are considered a utility breed for their fine eggs and meat. Although rare in the United States, they are gaining popularity on the Continent. They are not yet recognized by the APA, but their advocates are working to have them included in the Standard. Bantams are also popular in Europe but are on the ABA's Inactive list.

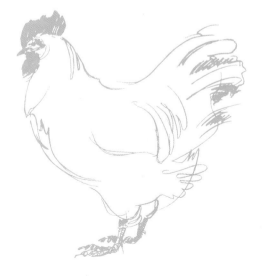

These Sulmtalers show the Golden Duckwing color pattern. Roosters are quite different from hens, but each has a small crest behind the comb. *Courtesy Greenfire Farms*

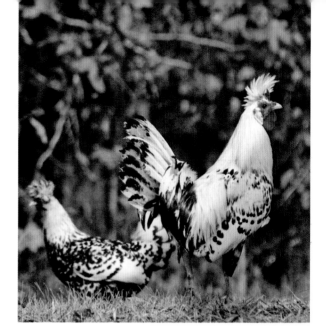

That feathery crest marks the Appenzeller Spitzhauben. It may look punk now, but in the past it suggested the white head coverings worn by the women of northeastern Switzerland. *Courtesy Greenfire Farms*

BRABANTER AND APPENZELLER SPITZHAUBEN

That pointed tuft on top of the head of these small chickens is like a pointed hood on both roosters and hens. Those with silvery white feathers tipped with black spangles glinting in the sun are Appenzeller Spitzhaubens. Those with three-lobed muffs and beards are *Brabanters*.

They have a V comb in front of the crest. The crest helps protect the comb from freezing in cold weather. They don't mind the weather, either hot and humid or cold and rainy. They eagerly chase bugs and enjoy their outdoor life. They tolerate confinement but would rather be out and about. They are kept as ornamental and exhibition birds for their unusual tufts and combs, but are good egg producers, too. They lay through the seasons, taking only a short break for molting.

Brabanters are chickens of Europe's Low Countries, the Brabant region of Belgium and the Netherlands. Artwork as far back as the seventeenth century provides documentation of heritage breed history. Appenzeller Spitzhaubens are Swiss. In German, the language of the Appenzell

region of Switzerland that these birds call home, Spitzhauben means pointed hood or bonnet. Local lore says their name comes from the resemblance of the crest to the lace bonnets that are traditional for women in that region.

Most Brabanters in the United States are Cream, an unrecognized color pattern of black spots on creamy feathers. Breeders also raise Gold Brabanters. Brabanters are not recognized by the APA.

Most Spitzhaubens in the United States are Silver Spangled, but fanciers are also raising the other traditional Swiss colors, Black and Gold Spangled. Other colors are being developed. Their advocates want all colors to be recognized by the APA, and are working toward that goal.

The ABA recognizes Brabanter and Spitzhauben bantams but hasn't seen any in a long time. Both are on the Inactive list. These breeds are already small, so bantams are indeed tiny.

SULTAN

These chickens are white feathery confections. From the crest, pure white behind a red horn comb, to the bearded and muffed face, pure white wings and tail, and white feathers that cover its legs and feet, this bird has always been a decorative accessory to regal life. As a practical chicken, hens lay white eggs.

Sultans were developed in Turkey and sent to England by an Englishman living there back in the nineteenth century. They arrived with the name Serai-Taook, meaning palace fowl, which has been translated as "Fowls of the Sultan." In a 1912 issue of *American Poultry Advocate*,

Judge W. E. Card describes them as having the large, globular crest of the Polish, the full abundant beard and whiskers of the Houdan, the feather-legs of the Cochin, the vulture hock of the booted bantams, the five toes of the Dorking, and the *V*-shaped comb of the La Fleche.

Their devotees preserve them, with occasional Houdan or Polish added to keep them vigorous and avoid inbreeding. Only white Sultans are recognized by the APA, but the ABA also recognizes Black and Blue bantams.

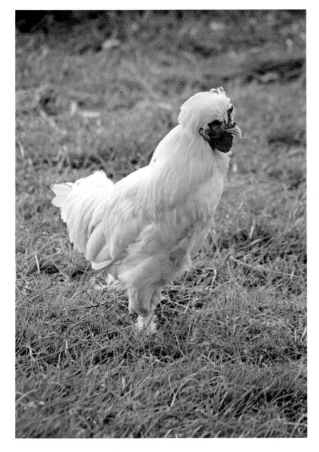

The Sultan is a chicken breed developed entirely as an ornament. It has all the fanciest points: a crest, muff and beard on the face, feathery legs, and five toes on each foot. As pretty as they are, they remain practical chickens who lay white eggs.
MikeLane45/Getty Images

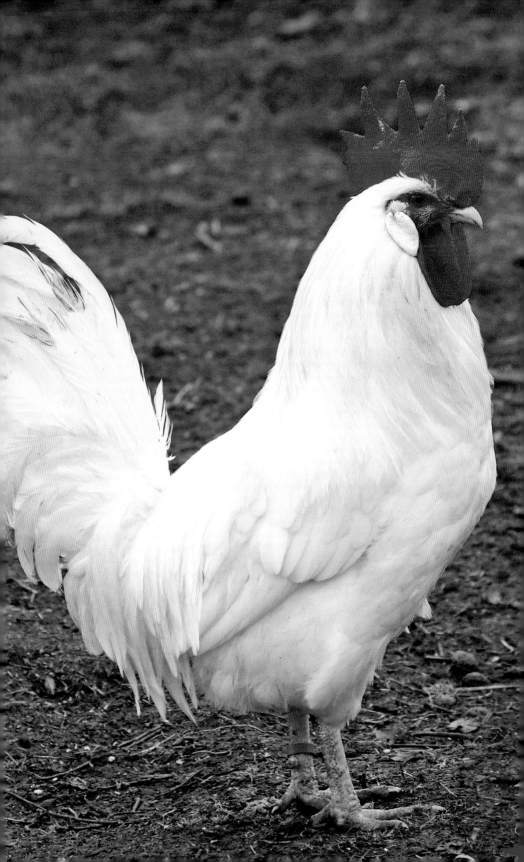

MEDITERRANEAN BREEDS

Mediterranean breeds are associated especially with Italy and Spain, warm climates with long histories of chicken breeding. They're egg breeds, known for regular and consistent egg production. They are more wiry in build than the dual-purpose breeds. They are non-sitting breeds, meaning that they do not get broody and will not hatch their own eggs. That trait was bred out over the years, as egg production ruled selective breeding.

Spanish, Minorcas, and Andalusians are recognized as separate breeds but share ancient roots in the Iberian Peninsula. They differ from Italian breeds in their white skin, leg color, and the genetics of white varieties. Black was their original plumage color. Development of these light Mediterranean egg breeds was influenced by English breeders in the nineteenth century with birds imported from Spain and Portugal.

Mediterranean countries were influenced by the religious conflicts of the Spanish Inquisition and the Protestant Reformation. Chicken breeding was not exempt from this influence: all breeds were by definition created by God. That precept was enforced by the Spanish Inquisition with torture and death, reducing the enthusiasm of breeders to take credit for a newly refined chicken breed.

Breeding for showing rather than production has reduced the remarkable egg-laying abilities of these breeds, but they are still the honored leaders. Commercially, Leghorns have become the sole American white egg producer.

All recognized Mediterranean breeds have white earlobes and lay white eggs, although Penedesencas are an exception and lay dark brown eggs.

There are no true bantams in this class. Leghorn bantams are among the most popular breeds shown, so develop your eye for bantam conformation watching them. Andalusian, Minorca, and White-Faced Black Spanish bantams are rarely seen. Catalana and Buttercup bantams are not known, if they were ever developed.

White Leghorns are a classic egg-laying breed. This dignified rooster presides over a backyard flock of hens that provide almost daily fresh eggs. Make friends with this neighbor to share their bounty. *Andrea Mangoni/ Shutterstock*

LEGHORN

Leghorns are often found in backyard flocks, even though standard Leghorns can be a bit high-strung, making them flighty around humans. Some settle down with attention. Leghorns are so popular that the APA recognizes sixteen different varieties, nine colors, and both rose and single combs. Fanciers raise others, such as Exchequer, a black and white Scottish variety.

Neither the comb nor the color will lead you to a correct identification for Leghorns. Check the size—Leghorn roosters grow only to about six pounds, hens to four and a half—and that distinctive tail, at 40 degrees from horizontal for roosters, a little lower at 35 degrees for hens.

Leghorns, with their yellow skin and prolific white eggs, originated in Italy. They take their name from the English version of the central Italy port city from which they were shipped, Livorno. Back in the nineteenth century, Italian egg-layers were popular all over Europe, but breeders focused on different qualities. In America, the Leghorn became "America's Business Hen" in the 1880s, setting it on the path to industrialization. Today, Leghorns have the most efficient feed-to-egg conversion ratio of all the Standard breeds, laying 225 to 250 eggs a year for seven years.

As a Mediterranean breed, Leghorns do best in warm climates. Single comb varieties are subject to freezing of comb and wattles in cold weather. Rose comb varieties don't have that problem. Summer heat doesn't bother them, although they need shade to escape direct sun.

Leghorns are so popular that both utility and exhibition strains are raised. In England, Leghorns are larger and have bigger combs and earlobes. Their tails are closely whipped, reflecting Minorca and Malay crossing, as compared to American Leghorns' lush, spreading tails. The APA devotes an entire page to variations on Leghorn combs in its 2010 Standard.

Both single and rose combs are recognized by the APA in Dark Brown, Light Brown, White, Buff, Black, and Silver. Single comb varieties in Red, Black-Tailed Red, Columbian, and Golden are recognized today. In 1884, the first Standard recognized only single comb white, black, and brown varieties. As breeders refined their flocks over the years, the brown variety was divided into Dark and Light, and the rose comb variety was added. Silver Duckwing, Golden Duckwing, and Silver varieties are also raised.

The ABA recognizes sixteen colors, including Exchequer, Barred, Blue, Buff Columbian, Dominique, Mille Fleur, and both comb types. Leghorn bantams are among the top ten most popular bantams shown.

This classic White Leghorn rooster is the patriarch of modern industrial layers. Leghorn hens are admired for their abundant egg laying. *Paulette Johnson/Fox Hill Photo*

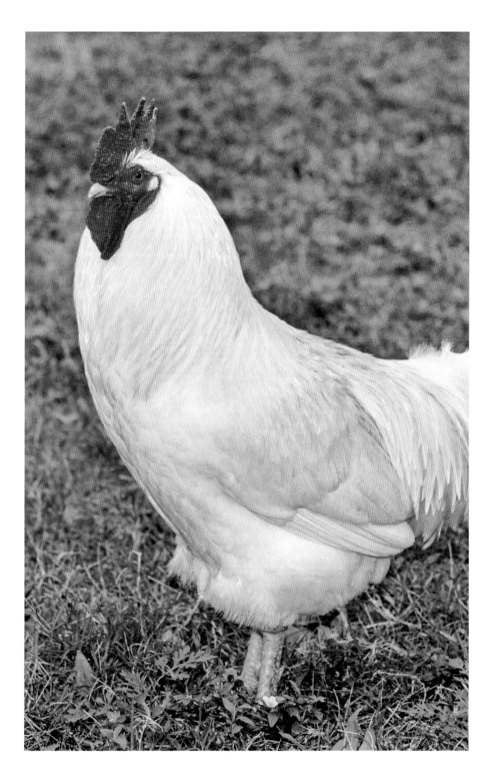

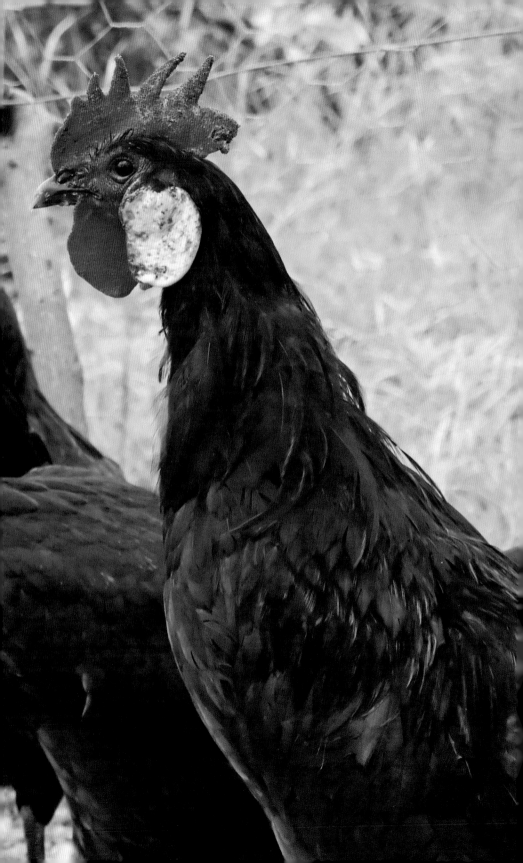

MINORCA

This big chicken may be black, white, or buff, but its face is red, rather than the white of its smaller Spanish cousin. The large earlobes are bright white, contrasting with the black or buff and blending in with the white. That big tail floats at a lower angle, just above the horizontal. It was known as a Red-Faced Spanish in the past, but now it is the Minorca.

Minorcas are usually found at poultry shows rather than in backyard flocks, but they are good layers. They have proven their strength and hardiness over the centuries. Minorcas were recognized as a separate breed, in Black and White Single Comb varieties, by the APA in 1888. Rose Comb Blacks and Rose Comb Whites were admitted later. The single comb can be a six-pointed masterpiece, standing up despite its formidable size. The hen's comb lops over properly.

That comb is a disadvantage in cold weather and can freeze, so breeders developed rose-comb Minorcas, retaining all their fine qualities but adding the compact comb by crossing them with Hamburgs.

The Minorca's history was influenced by British colonial wars. The first poultry show that had a class for Minorcas was in 1853 at Bristol, England. Minorcas caught on with breeders twenty-five years later, and a few were imported to the United States around 1885.

The Single Comb Buff was also recognized. Single Comb Buffs were the result of adding Buff Leghorns and Brahmas, part of the buff color craze of the late nineteenth century. Leg color varies with plumage.

Minorcas are nine pounds for roosters, seven and a half for hens. Size is an important qualification. Breeders who tried to add size by breeding Langshans or Orpingtons were disappointed, and the original silvery-black plumage is now greenish black as a result of those cross-breeding efforts.

The ABA recognizes single and rose comb Black, Buff, Self Blue, and White bantams. That long back can look odd on a bantam but gives them a majestic carriage.

Minorcas are big chickens, with red faces rather than the white of their White-Faced Black Spanish cousins. The hens' combs are so large, they flop over. *Thomas Crawford/Getty Images*

WHITE-FACED BLACK SPANISH

A distinctive white face instantly identifies this breed as a White-Faced Black Spanish. That white face is a beacon against the black feathers, topped off by bright red comb and wattles.

The white skin should be smooth, but some folding is inevitable. Size is more desired than smoothness. The white face should be longer than the red wattles on both males and females, but hens have smaller faces than males. Cold weather can mar the perfection of their white faces with dark spots. These are birds that naturally incline to a warm Mediterranean climate.

These are somewhat leggier than the other Mediterranean breeds, and their necks stretch up a bit longer, too. They are larger than Leghorns, Anconas, and Andalusians, but smaller than Minorcas. White-Faced Black Spanish have dark legs with pink on the bottoms of their feet, compared with the yellow legs of the Italian Leghorns. Roosters have graceful tails, carried at a 45-degree angle.

Their large chalk-white eggs have distinguished them on both sides of the Atlantic. They were a popular breed in early America, cited in 1816 as one of the true breeds then. Because they take their time to mature and require extra care to prepare for the show ring, they are now a rare but wonderful backyard sighting.

They are the oldest breed of the Mediterranean class, the ancestor of white egg chickens. Records are few, but the white face was firmly established by around 1600. White-Faced Black Spanish were probably developed from Castilian chickens with red faces and white earlobes in the seventeenth century. Their meat is also highly recommended, as white and flavorful.

White Spanish with white faces have existed in the past, but they are not formally recognized. The contrast of color is less dramatic, but they have all the other fine qualities of this honored breed. The ABA recognizes a Blue variety as well as Black.

Bantams grow faster than their large fowl correlates. Large fowl may not be as large as they should be, and bantams not as small. High protein feed is recommended for large fowl chicks, to get them growing well.

The name White-Faced Black Spanish describes the distinctive feature of this rooster. He may appear unusual, but he represents an ancient breed, valued for chalk-white eggs. *Paulette Johnson/Fox Hill Photo*

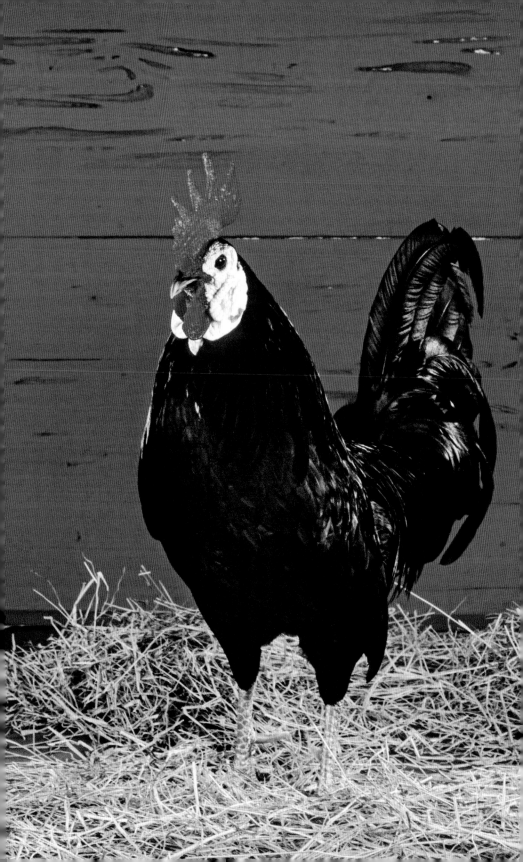

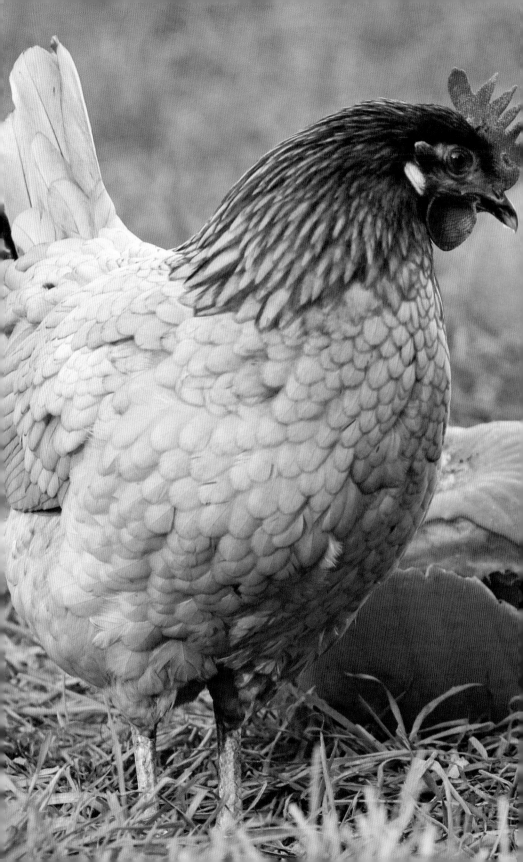

ANDALUSIAN

Andalusians take their name from a province in Spain. They aren't the only blue chicken, but they are the best known for their misty bluish gray plumage, the only color variety for which they are recognized. They are larger than their Leghorn cousins in the Mediterranean class at seven pounds for a rooster, five and a half pounds for a hen.

Blue Andalusians were first imported to England in the mid-nineteenth century and excited such interest that Splash and Blue cocks were being bred to any black hen even remotely resembling Spanish type to meet the demand. The attraction was perhaps irresistible: unusual, eye-catching, and difficult to get right or reproduce. Blue Andalusians were in that original 1874 Standard, even if not many breeders were successfully keeping them.

Blue, also called slate and gray, chickens were common in England, so Spanish breeds were often crossed with blue Games and other breeds. Blue Andalusians of today are actually the Blue Laced color pattern, blue feathers with a darker blue edging around the feather, as compared with Self Blue, which is an even shade of blue all over.

The blue color never breeds true, for genetic reasons. Breeding blue to blue produces approximately one-quarter black, one-quarter splash and half blue offspring. Breeding Splash to Black results in all blue offspring, but the color quality is washed out, not the vibrant blue with contrasting lacing that is the esteemed ideal. The darkest hens breed the best blue laced offspring.

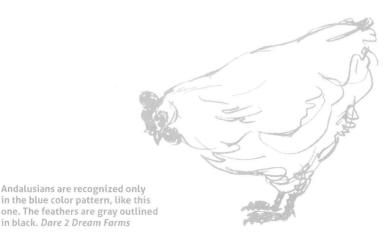

Andalusians are recognized only in the blue color pattern, like this one. The feathers are gray outlined in black. *Dare 2 Dream Farms*

ANCONA

Black feathers gleam glossy green in the sunlight, flashing *V*-shaped white tips on the feathers. They are small but not bantams. This flock, each head topped with a bright red comb and white earlobes, and standing on bright yellow legs, are Anconas.

They take their name from the port city Ancona on Italy's east coast, across from the western region of Tuscany where Leghorns developed. Anconas are so similar to Leghorns that they are sometimes called Mottled Leghorns, but they've been a separate breed for more than a century, and were recognized as such by the APA in 1898. The rose comb variety was recognized in 1914.

Anconas are known as excellent layers, which may have encouraged breeders to develop the rose comb variety so they can be kept in colder climates. They are active, and good foragers. Their advocates in the late nineteenth century found them so hardy that they were able to sustain themselves on open range in wet, windswept conditions that had overwhelmed all other breeds. The downside of that hardiness is a high-strung temperament. While Leghorns are described as flighty, Anconas are called pheasant, suggesting that they are almost wild. However, while Ancona hens can be wary and move very fast, they fit in with a mixed flock well.

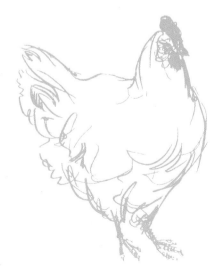

This Italian Ancona is similar to a Leghorn and equally revered for its eggs. This rooster presides over hens whose combs flop over rather than standing up straight like his. Keep them in your yard for plenty of fresh white eggs.
Erni/Shutterstock

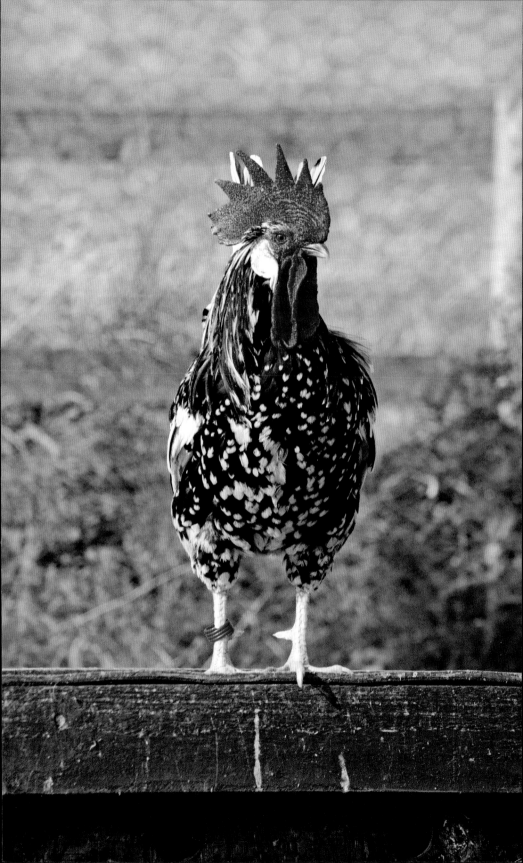

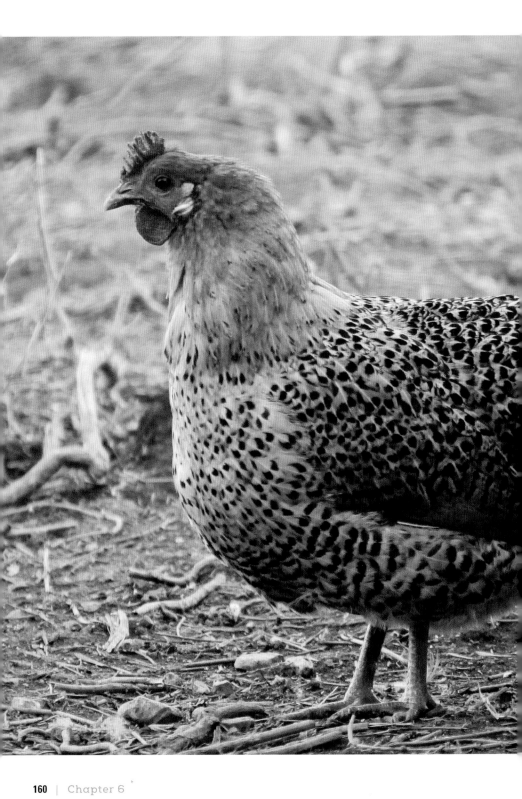

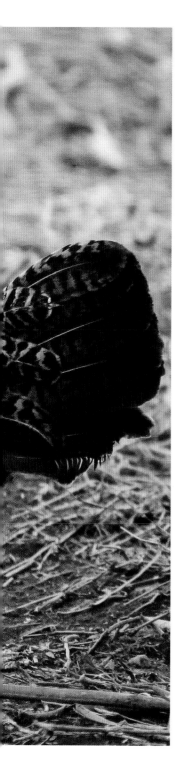

SICILIAN BUTTERCUP

A cup-shaped comb distinctively crowns the head of the Sicilian Buttercup. Although the Standard accepts their origin as Sicily, Buttercups were more likely developed by Arabs of North Africa, who traveled through the Mediterranean countries. The chickens of North Africa are smaller than the Sicilian Buttercup, with a smaller comb. Buttercups have more than a passing resemblance to Egyptian Fayoumis. Buttercups could have been influenced by the Leghorns after they arrived in Italy, getting bigger and enhancing that kingly crown.

Buttercups were first imported to the United States in 1835 and accepted into the Standard of Perfection in 1918. Those willow green legs are elusive for breeders, but without them, Buttercups are disqualified from being shown. Chicks' legs are yellowish until they develop the slate color at four to six months of age. At that age, the greenish tint will also develop.

The comb must stand straight, not flop over, and not have a third row of points. The required coloring can be just as difficult to breed as the correct comb and leg tone. The ideal rooster has a brilliant red comb complemented by a light horn beak topping his orange head and lustrous reddish orange feathers flowing down to his back. His cape should have black spangles and his black tail glisten green. Hens are golden buff with little points of black within the feathers.

The hens often develop spurs. That's not uncommon on Mediterranean breeds, but it's not acceptable in the show ring.

Like other Mediterranean breeds, they are non-sitters. They are an egg production breed and lay white eggs. Exhibition weights top out at six and a half pounds for males and five pounds for females.

They live up to their reputation as a flighty breed, but if they are handled daily from the time they hatch, they can be tame around people. When they are trained with treats such as sunflower seeds, they will come forward to greet visitors.

If you spot any bantams of this breed, notify the local bantam fanciers! None have been seen in a long time and this bantam may be headed for Inactive status.

The Sicilian Buttercup has a unique crown comb. They have a musical trill rather than a cackle. *Dare 2 Dream Farms*

CATALANA

This large golden rooster has a green tail, with green and buff sickle feathers flowing toward it. Golden hens have black tails. If they flap their wings, you will see flashes of black on them.

Their full Spanish name, Catalana del Prat Leonada, takes the name of its country, Catalonia, the area around Barcelona, Spain, and the farming district where it was developed, El Prat de Llobregat.

Catalanas are one of the large Mediterranean breeds, valued for their meat as well as their eggs. Although they are a rare sighting in North America, they are popular in South America. Catalanas came on the official poultry scene at the 1902 World's Fair in Madrid, Spain. They had been developed over the nineteenth century from local landrace chickens and larger Cochins or other Asiatic breeds. They are probably not related to the local Lmpordanesa and Penedesenca, both of which lay dark brown eggs. Catalanas lay white eggs. They have noticeable white earlobes, as the other Spanish breeds do.

Catalanas do best outdoors, where they can forage for themselves and use their energy in productive scratching. They do well in hot weather. A chicken for the warm, sunny days of Spain is now a good though infrequent choice for American backyards.

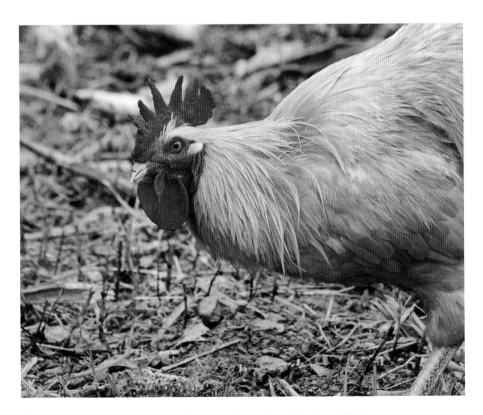

Catalanas enjoy warm weather, as befits a breed from Spain. A backyard flock will gives its keepers plenty of large, white eggs. *Terry Wild Stock*

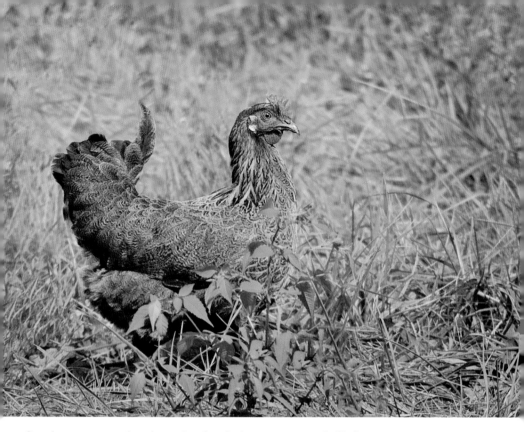

Penedesencas are good egg layers, but they don't warm up to people. Their attention is focused on foraging and taking care of chicken business. They are cold hardy and don't mind snow. *Rina Marie Ricketts/Faithful with Little Farm*

PENEDESENCA

Check out those combs. Penedesencas have a mass of side sprigs at the back of the single comb, or it may look like a cross from above, with one large sprig sticking out from each side.

Side sprigs, which are extra points sticking out from the comb, are unacceptable in recognized breeds. The comb starts as a single comb but expands into several lobes at the rear. In the Catalan language this is called a "carnation comb" *(cresta en clavell)* or a "king's comb."

Penedesencas are related to another brown egg–laying Spanish, Empordanesas, but only the Penedesenca has been brought to the United States. Emporadanesas have the expected red earlobes. They are more like Catalanas, buff with contrasting tails— either black, blue, or white.

The breed disappeared from public view during the upheaval of the Spanish Civil War and World War II. They have been championed by some breeders, so you may see them foraging in a backyard flock.

Penedesencas are unusual in that they lay dark brown eggs despite their white earlobes. Their eggs are so dark as to be nearly black, especially those laid by young hens. They are hardy and appreciated for their meat as well as their eggs. They may be black, wheaten partridge, or crele, a variation of Black Breasted Red coloring with barring on the feathers. Roosters grow to six and a half pounds, and hens weigh about four and a half pounds.

Penedesencas are not recognized by the APA, and there are no bantams.

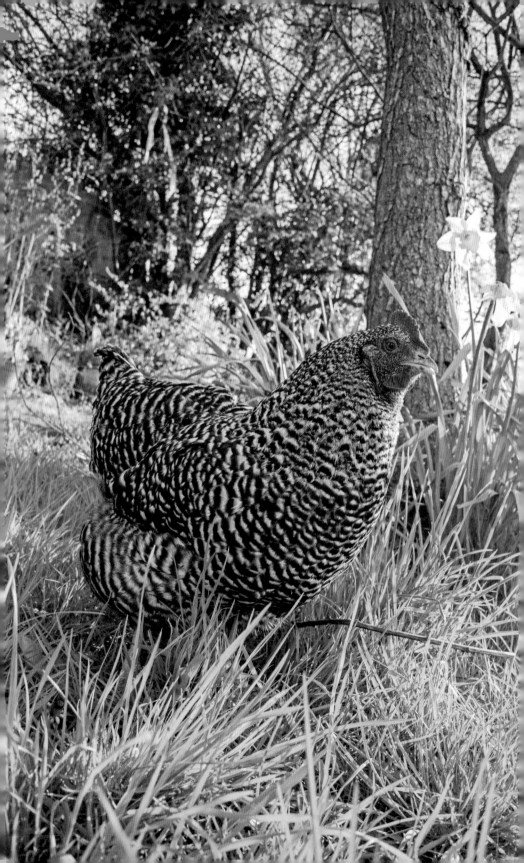

CONTINENTAL BREEDS

The Continental class carries a whiff of the Grand Tour expeditions taken by upper-class young English men across the Channel to the Netherlands, France, Germany, and other European countries. The name stays with chickens that trace their roots back to those countries today.

They are subdivided into Northern European, including Barnevelders, Campines, Hamburgs, Lakenvelders, and Welsummers; Polish, a class for one breed alone; and French, which include Houdans, Crèvecoeurs, La Fleche, and Faverolles. Both large fowl and bantams are kept. They reflect their climate conditions, ranging from the cool and wet north to the milder French countryside. (The Crested Breeds that are exhibited in these categories have their own section in this book.)

Continental breeds are varied and colorful. Their history as barnyard stalwarts keeping the farm family in eggs and meat is expressed today in their distinctive appearance and feathering. They have crests and unusual combs. Bantams show muffs, beards, and boots.

Several of the Continental breeds are well known and often seen, but others have declined to the point of being rare sightings.

Continental breeds are often named for the locales with which they are associated. Their names follow the geography and history of their development across Europe, reminding Americans that these breeds carry international intrigue with their feathers.

Two major wars on the European continent affected all these breeds. Many flocks were decimated when their starving owners had no other choice but to eat them. Support for breeds with German roots was undermined by distaste for all things associated with German history.

Breeds that survived now hold that history as part of their past. Remote locations that were not as severely affected by the war maintained their flocks, an important aspect of recovery from the devastation. White eggs remain the classic color laid by these breeds. The white eggs that were once most desirable to consumers are now less preferred than brown and other colors, adding to the decline of these breeds.

The grass hides this Marans chicken's legs. The French Marans have feathered legs, but English Marans have clean (no feathers) legs. Her cuckoo feathers, the black-and-white pattern, has a long history and camouflages chickens in dappled sunlight. *Caz Harris Photography/Shutterstock*

BARNEVELDER

This chicken appears so dark as to be almost black in the shade, but its feathers shine with a blue-green sheen in the sunlight. Hens and roosters both feature five-pointed combs and yellow legs.

Their feather pattern is Double Laced, with two black stripes at the edges of each reddish brown feather. In the United States, only the Double Laced variety of Barnvelders is recognized by the APA, although the United Kingdom and The Netherlands recognize other colors.

Barnevelders were developed at the early twentieth century for their dark brown eggs, but the feather color was so exceptional that it became another desirable attribute. Their color and active disposition help them avoid predators as they forage on pasture.

Barneveld, a Dutch town east of Utrecht, was becoming the hub of the Netherlands' egg business in the late nineteenth century. The region sold a lot of eggs to England, and large dark brown eggs commanded a premium price. Crossing the local dark egg layers with breeds such as the white-egg-laying Cornish risked the dark egg color that was so prized, so the arrival of the brown egg laying Cochins, Brahmas, and Langshans from China in the mid-1800s advanced the development of this breed.

One breeder imported some birds that were prototypes of Gold Laced Wyandottes from the United States in 1898 to add to his Barnevelders. After the turn of the century, Buff Orpingtons were added. Barnevelders were admitted to the APA Standard in 1991, and although Barnevelder bantams were developed, they are Inactive in the United States.

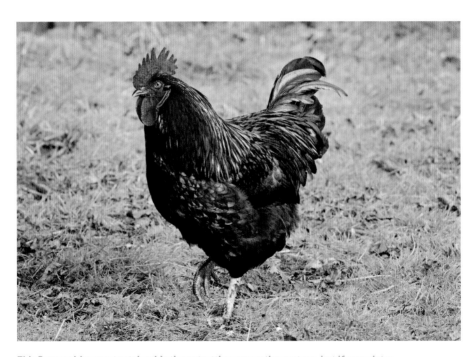

This Barnevelder rooster takes his time strutting across the pasture, but if a predator appears, he'll lead his flock in a wild escape. Their zig-zag running keeps them out of predators' talons. *Chrislofotos/Shutterstock*

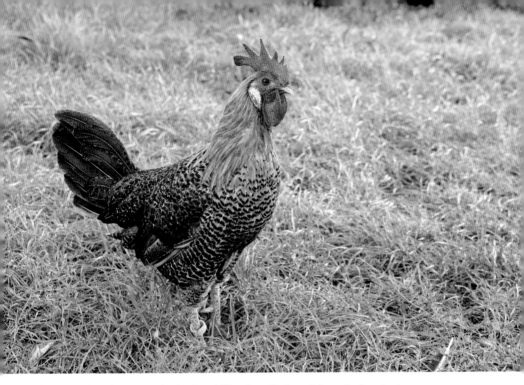

This Golden Campine rooster looks almost like a hen. He doesn't have the long back and tail feathers most roosters do. He's no less masculine, though, and is a good leader for a backyard flock. *Erni/Shutterstock*

CAMPINE

Campine roosters and hens both have solid-color heads, either golden bay or white, over the barred feathers that cover the rest of the body. Their sharp eyes are brown, not the reddish bay of Leghorns.

Roosters are henny feathered, meaning that they don't have the showy sickle feathers in the tail or the long hackle and saddle feathers on their backs, giving them a different silhouette.

Notice their similarities to Fayoumis and their relatives, the Buttercup. This breed likely arrived in Europe via Africa, although other reports suggest it came overland from the Middle East. Campines trace their roots back to Belgium. They are similar to Braekels, a larger version with roosters that have different plumage from hens. Belgian breeders preferred the white

hackles and black tails of Braekel roosters, but British breeders settled on the overall barred plumage for both roosters and hens in 1902.

One of the newly acquired henny feathered Silver Campines received major awards at a 1904 English show, and all Campine breeders sought his sons for their flocks.

Their original purpose was to lay plentiful white eggs, for which they are still revered. Few are shown, although their unusual plumage makes them a draw at poultry shows. They have never been numerous and had to be readmitted to the Standard after the breed was dropped in 1989 for lack of participation.

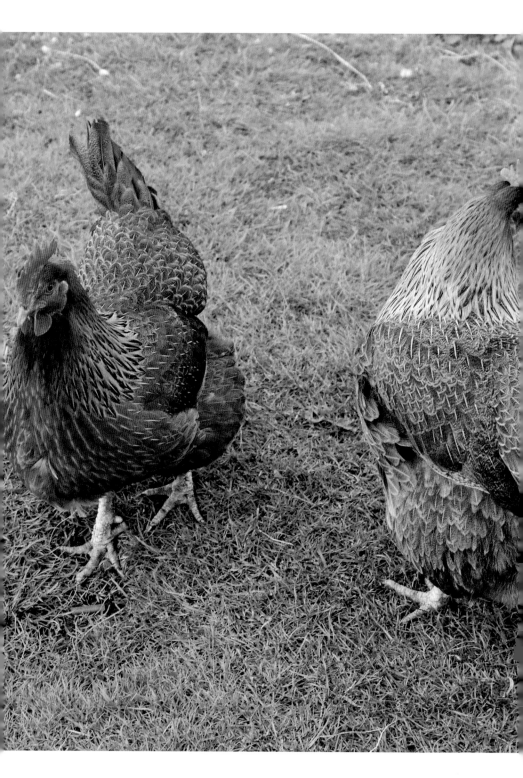

WELSUMMER

Dappled shades of brown catch the sunlight on these chickens. The rooster sports a black tail behind a golden head and back, but the girls are all colors of brown with bits of black and gray. Eggs in the nest box are terra cotta brown, some with speckles. They are Welsummers.

Those rich brown eggs were the original goal of developing this breed, back in the late nineteenth century in the Netherlands. Chicken keepers in the small town of Welsum, near Barneveld, wanted those dark brown eggs from their chickens. Like Barnevelders, the original birds were a mixed group, because their breeders were more interested in the color of the eggs than developing a reliable, reproducible breed. They bred those dark-brown-egg laying Langshans into their flocks, which already had the long legs and neck of their Malay influence and some partridge coloration from other Asiatics. The gene for blue feathers showed up in some. Flock keepers breeding nearby Barnevelders swapped chickens from their flocks.

All that mixing affected the dark brown eggs that were the original goal. The hens who laid the most eggs and started laying early in the spring laid lighter eggs than the girls who started laying later. Egg production was declining even before Welsummers got established.

Adding Rhode Island Reds, which lay brown eggs, and Brown or Partridge Leghorns, white egg layers, to the flocks improved egg production and gave them more uniform red-brown color but also lightened that desirable dark brown egg color. By this time, World War I was disrupting life in Europe, but sturdy egg layers such as the Welsummer contributed to feeding the devastated nations.

Welsummers made their way to the United States, their dark eggs causing comment where ever they went. Their color pattern is sometimes called red partridge, although that's unofficial. No breeders championed their cause as an exhibition bird at that time. They were eventually recognized in the Standard in 1991. The APA Standard notes that their egg laying ability should be considered in judging them at shows. Welsummer bantams are on the Inactive list.

Their Rhode Island Red heritage shows in their flat back, and the Barnevelder in the way they carry their tails high. Chicks are to some extent auto-sexing, that is, males and females look different from the start. Females are darker and more clearly marked and have a stripe behind the eye. Males are lighter, with less distinct markings and a spot behind the eye. It's a judgment call, not as definitive as sex-linked birds of entirely different colors, but a distinction that makes the Welsummer special.

These busy Welsummer hens lay dark brown eggs, sometimes speckled. The Welsummer is a composite breed that became popular in the early twentieth century. I can tell which of my Welsummers laid those distinctive eggs. *Linda Steward/Getty Images*

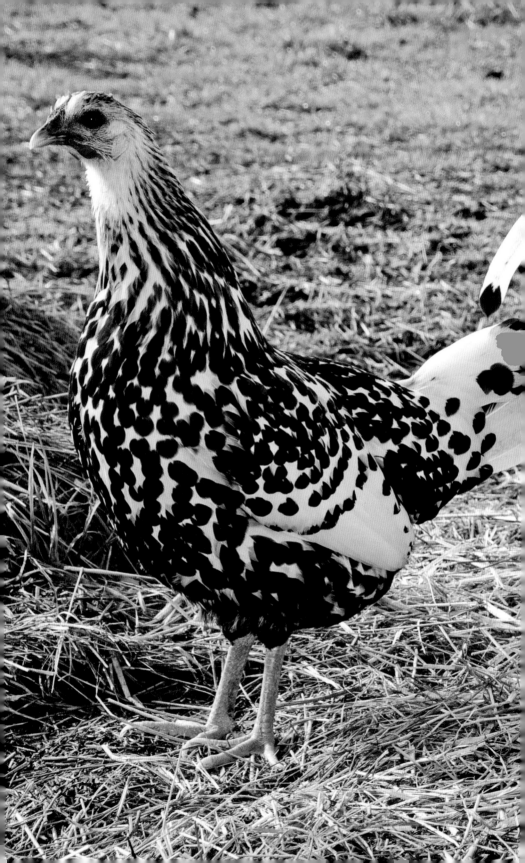

HAMBURG

These chickens are small and graceful on their blue legs. Some are solid white or black, but others have penciled white or gold feathers and still others have larger black markings called spangles. Careful of their long tails! Their feathers are close to their bodies, and their heads are crowned with rose combs. They are similar to Leghorns, but smaller. Their legs are shorter, giving them a fuller appearance than the long, slender Leghorn. Hamburgs have shorter, straighter backs leading to less lush tails.

The name Hamburg encompasses chickens that descended from varied origins. The English poultry judge who gave them that name in 1850 knew them well as northern English chickens but chose to call them Hamburgs because he thought that they were originally imported from the city of that name. Lancashire Mooneys, so called for the large spangles that were like moons on their feathers, and Yorkshire Pheasant Fowl were two of the local breeds that became the Black and Spangled Hamburgs. The name was attacked at the time as confusing these English chickens with Brabanters and other spangled, bearded, and crested breeds.

Dutch chickens were in the mix, antecedents of the penciled varieties.

One expert considers that today, with the popularity of Hamburgs, the penciled varieties could be separated out from the spangled and solid colors and given a Dutch name, Hollandse Hoen. Penciled and White Hamburgs tend to be smaller than the other varieties.

Feather markings are important in this penciled and spangled breed. The spangle is the black teardrop at the end of the feather, against the silver or gold of the rest of the feather. Penciled feathers have straight black lines across them. In Silver Penciled Hamburgs, the rooster is all white on his head, neck, breast, and part of his wings, with penciling only on some wing feathers. His tail is black, with white edges. Hens have white heads but are otherwise penciled all over.

Their white eggs are medium size, not commercially competitive with large Leghorn eggs. Hamburgs were prized for their eggs in the past.

As active as they are, they tolerate confinement. They don't mind cold weather, and those rose combs don't freeze.

All six currently recognized varieties were in the first Standard in 1874. Bantams are also recognized in all six varieties.

This Silver Spangled Hamburg shows the large black spangles on white feathers. Golden Spangled Hamburgs have black spangles on golden feathers. They are smaller than Leghorns but, like them, are good layers. *Amy McNabb/Shutterstock*

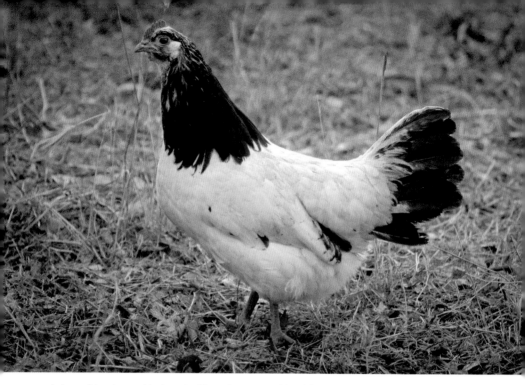

Lakenvelders have a black-and-white color pattern identified with the city of Lakervelt in the Dutch/German border region. Cattle, hogs, and rabbits that trace their ancestry to that region share white against black colors. *Dare 2 Dream Farms*

LAKENVELDER

Lakenvelders are stark black and white chickens, topped with a bright red comb and wattles. Both roosters and hens have intense black necks and capes over white shoulders, followed by a black tail. It's a difficult color pattern to breed, with white feathers frequently showing up in the black areas, and vice versa.

They look like a small black and white Leghorn. Even large fowl Lakenvelders are small, and Lakenvelder bantams are tiny, but they are good egg layers.

They are active foragers, but their bright white feathers make them a target for predators on pasture. A better place for them is on a farm, with its orchards, gardens, and farm buildings. They are wary and don't warm up to people as fast as calmer breeds.

They take their name from the Dutch town of Lakervelt near the German border with Westfalen, northern Rheinland, and Hannover. According to the *1910 Encyclopedia of Poultry*, the breed had nearly died out in the previous century but was revived to become the most popular breed in Germany. But that German name and heritage contributed to lost popularity after World War I.

The APA recognized Lakenvelders in 1939, as Europe was wracked again by war. The breed has recovered in Europe better than it has in England or the United States.

KRAIENKOPPE

The birds in this breed have the powerful look of country chickens, like Games. Kraienkoppe carry their red-earlobed heads high, over a wide tail. Tight feathers give them a sleek look.

They lay plentiful medium to small white or tinted eggs, an exception to the rule that earlobe color reflects egg color. The hens make good broody hens and good mothers.They are protective of their chicks and will fight to defend them.

Historically, Kraienkoppe come from the German/Dutch border region, in the East Dutch province of Twente. Germans call them Kraienkoppen, but in The Netherlands, Dutch keepers call them Twentse, and Kraienkoppes are another breed entirely. Confused?

The Kraienkoppe was derived from the Pheasant Malay, an Oriental Game. Belgian Game, Dutch landraces, and Leghorns are also in their background. In the past, they were used for cock fighting.

They retain an independent spirit, eager to get up into the trees and range free. That strength and wandering disposition makes them less likely to be backyard pets, but they are a good practical bird for the small homestead. They fly well. They are hardy and seldom succumb to any illness. They don't mind the cold and lay well through cold weather.

The Kraienkoppe was recognizable as a breed in Europe in the early 1800s. Here in the United States the Kraienkoppe is not recognized by the APA. Kraienkoppes were recognized in the German Standard in 1926.

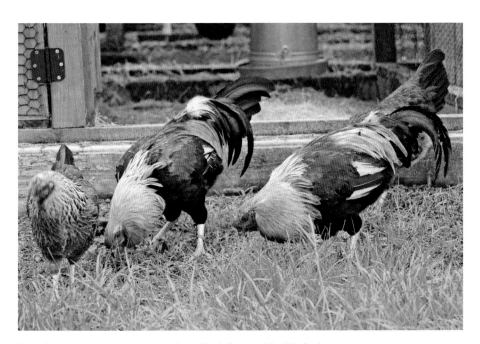

Note the compact walnut comb on these Black-Breasted Red Kraienkoppe roosters. They are powerful country chickens who can protect themselves on free range. They may fly out of the backyard and are wary of people. *Courtesy Greenfire Farms*

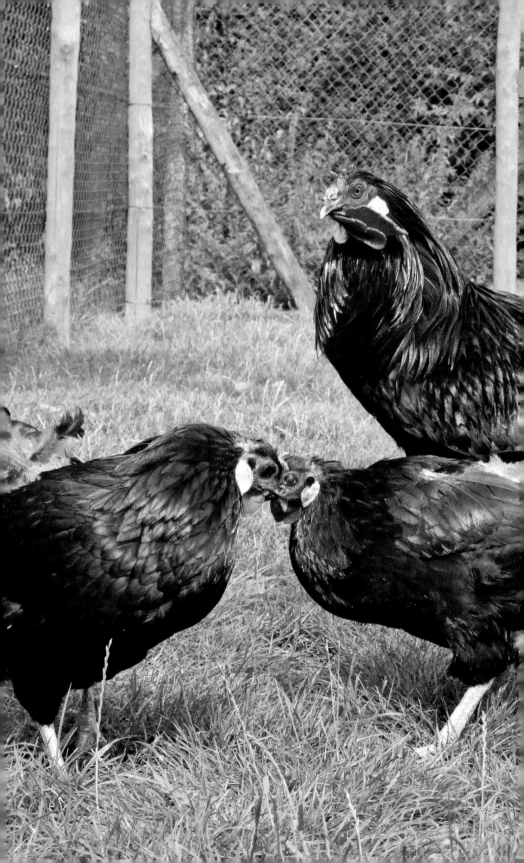

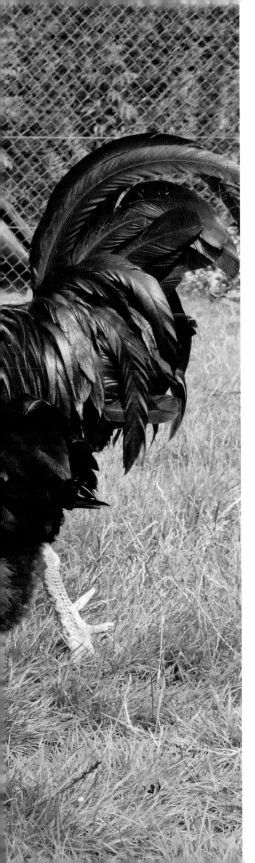

LA FLECHE

The bright red *V*-shaped horn comb stands out on the La Fleche. It doesn't have the crest of its French relatives, the Crèvecoeur and the Houdan.

The La Fleche, probably the oldest member of the French class, was selected and managed for egg and meat production in Britain and North America. Its meat is white and highly prized, but La Fleche grow slowly, discouraging producers who want to turn their flocks into cash quickly.

The La Fleche take their name from the town of La Fleche, around which production was centered in the early nineteenth century. Their actual history goes much farther back, to the fifteenth century or even earlier. Confusion over names given to local fowl makes it difficult to trace their history. They probably resulted from crossing Polish, Crèvecoeur, and Spanish birds, which gave them their white earlobes.

They have sometimes been called "the Horned Fowl." Although now clean-headed, some breeders report occasional offspring with small crests or tassels. The French standard requires a crest. La Fleche have glossy greenish black feathers and prominent combs with nicely rounded points. They should have strong, well-spaced rangy legs, broad shoulders, full breasts, and long, broad backs sloping downward from shoulder to tail.

They are recognized only in black, but in the past other colors were popular. In 1580, Prudens Choiselat wrote in *A Discourse of Housebandrie* that blacks, reds, and tawny were the best. Blue and white strains have existed in the more recent past.

The two-pronged horn comb is distinctive of these French La Fleche chickens. Some call them Horned Fowl. Their black feathers gleam iridescent green in the sun, and hens lay eggs as white as their earlobes. *Courtesy of the Livestock Conservancy*

FAVEROLLES

This chicken's legs are feathered but without covering the feet, and the rooster's plumage is a patchwork of contrast, from the black muffs and beard on his light yellow head and neck to his straw yellow sickles over a black tail. Hens are a warm salmon brown with white fluffy faces. They've all got that fifth toe.

Faverolles are a French breed developed from local Houdans, Asiatic stock, and the Dorking. The muff is often attributed to the Houdan, but some strains of Dorkings were muffed when Faverolles were developed in the late nineteenth century. Named after a French town, the final *S* is correct in the singular.

They are known for laying through cold weather, and are large bodied and make a good meat breed. Today, Houdans, Crèvecoeurs, and Faverolles are all about the same size.

The Houdan-Asiatic crosses were popular with the English poultry market, but French breeders didn't much care what color they were or what kind of comb they had, so in England, the breed needed to be refined into a standard description. They now have single combs and lay light brown eggs.

Faverolles are the only APA-recognized breed with the Salmon color variety, a silver wheaten pattern, which is very different on cocks and hens. Hens may show lacing on their salmon feathers, which does not disqualify them. The male looks very much like a Dark Dorking, and females are similar to wheaten game hens. The APA also recognizes White in large fowl and bantams, but the ABA recognizes Black, Blue, and Buff as well.

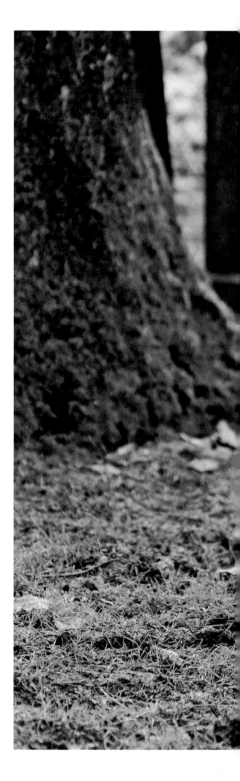

The Salmon Faverolles hen has a fluffy face, with a beard and muffs even covering her earlobes. Faverolles are the only breed recognized in the Salmon color variety. They lay light brown eggs. *Andyworks/Getty Images*

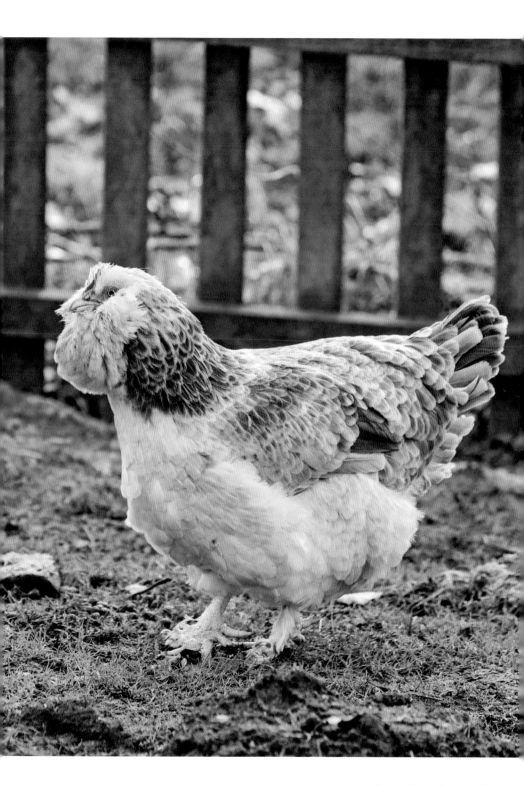

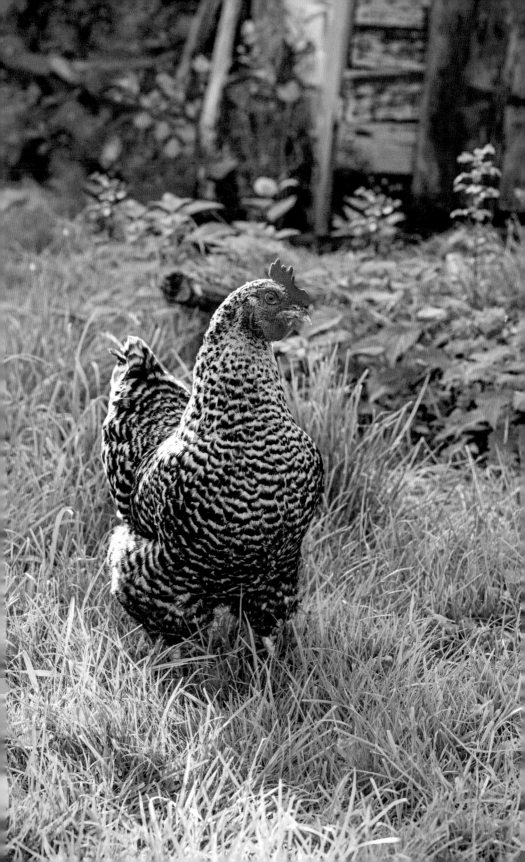

MARANS

While there are some feathers on Marans' legs, but they are more like a game chicken than Asiatic breeds. Their feathers are neatly folded, smooth and close to the body. They have white skin and legs, but red earlobes indicate that they lay brown eggs.

Marans were developed in the area around the small town of Marans, France. Although the final *S* isn't pronounced in French, it's part of the correct spelling, even in the English singular. It's not far from the coastal city of La Rochelle, so imported chickens from other parts of the world had long influenced local flocks. Marans barnyards had a lot of Asian and English game chicken influence, making them strong, with close, hard feathers.

When Asiatic chickens arrived in the nineteenth century, their brown eggs and larger size made them an obvious choice to add to brown-egg-laying flocks. Black Langshan breeders in the area were the origin of the birds that were eventually refined into Marans, and their Black Copper color.

The dark brown color of the eggs is an important breed qualification. To be in good standing as a Marans, hens must lay eggs of at least a Number 4 on a color chart ranging from 1, a white egg, through 9, nearly black.

Those dark brown eggs were the most important feature for breeders who initially worked with them in the late nineteenth century. They weren't concerned if their hens had feathers on their legs or not, or if they weren't completely black. That led to separate strains: English Marans have clean legs. French Marans have feathered legs. When American breeders determined to form a breed club in 2007 and pursue formal APA recognition, they chose to follow the French standard of feathered legs.

Marans are the latest addition to the French subclass of Continental breeds. Black Copper and Wheaten varieties were admitted to the Standard in 2011. White was added in 2014. Black Copper is also a new color pattern, recognized in no other breed. Black Copper roosters are black with bright copper heads, backs, and other accent feathers. The green shine from their black tails contrasts brightly with the warm copper head and back. Hens are similar, but less showy with less copper.

Breeders who campaigned to achieve recognition of three colors in four years continue to work with other colors of their beloved breed: Cuckoo, Blue, Blue Copper, Blue Wheaten, Birchen, Black-Tailed Buff, Cuckoo, Columbian (called Ermine in France), and Salmon.

This Cuckoo Marans is a popular color but not yet recognized for the show ring. Instead, find Cuckoo Marans in backyards, where their keepers have bragging rights on their dark brown eggs. *Caz Harris Photography/Shutterstock*

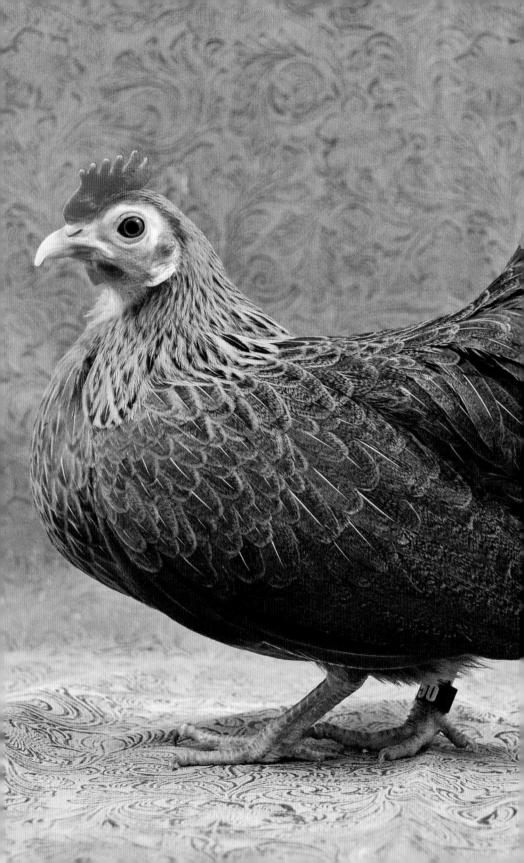

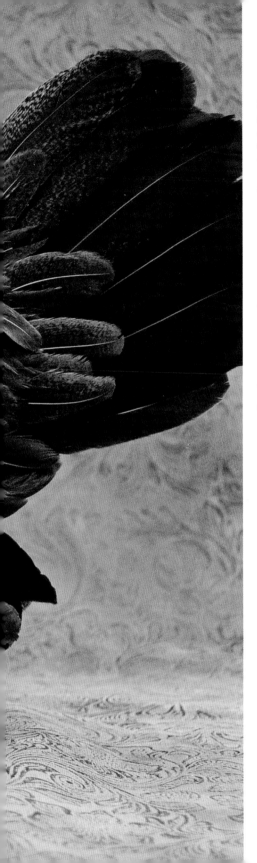

DUTCH

Sickle feathers gracefully flow off the small Dutch chickens' backs, and their tails extend out behind them. Their single comb with five distinct points clearly separates them from Rosecomb bantams.

These true bantams are popular, and ten color varieties are recognized. You may see Black, Blue, Blue Light Brown, Cuckoo, Golden, Light Brown, Cream Light Brown, Blue Cream Light Brown, Self Blue, Silver, Wheaten, or White Dutch bantams, recognized by the ABA. The APA recognizes six color varieties. Fanciers raise them in many other colors, so don't be distracted if you see a Red-Shouldered White or Mille Fleur. Dutch bantams are shown in the Single Comb Clean Legged class.

Dutch bantams have a long history, possibly developed from the small Red Junglefowl and other small Indonesian chickens brought back to the Netherlands. They were noted at The Hague Zoo in 1882 but didn't make their way to America until the 1950s. Imports in the 1970s introduced them to more fanciers, who formed the American Dutch Bantam Society in 1986.

Ideally, this Dutch bantam hen's comb would have only five distinct points. This variation doesn't disqualify her from being shown, and it would never be noticed in a backyard flock. Dutch bantams are frequently shown in any of ten color varieties. *Courtesy of the Livestock Conservancy*

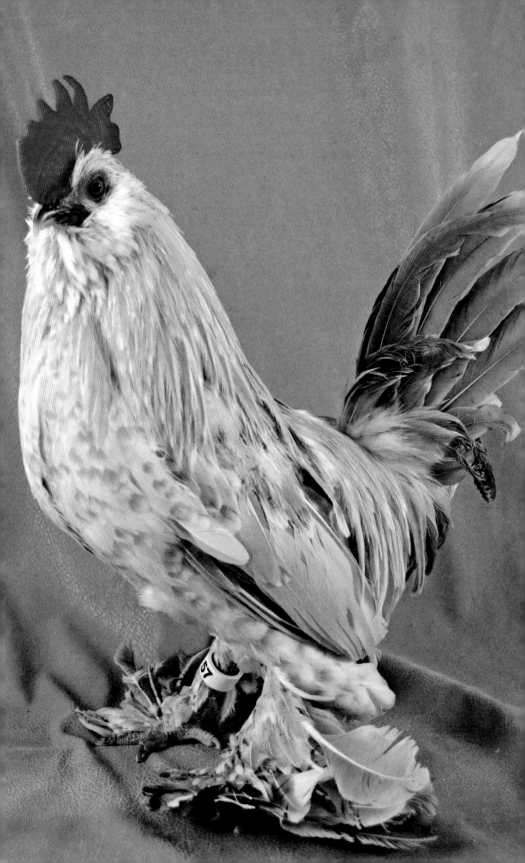

BOOTED, BELGIAN BEARDED D'ANVERS AND D'UCCLE

These chickens carry their long tails high and their wings low. If seen outdoors, they may be on fine sand or well-trimmed grass, to protect their feathers. Keeping the feathers clean and unbroken is a priority for winning at the shows.

Booted, Belgian Bearded d'Anvers, and Belgian Bearded d'Uccle are related and similar but differentiated by feathered feet, muffs and beards, and comb type. Booted have a single comb and no beard. The d'Anvers has muffs and beard and rose combs but clean legs. The d'Uccle has muffs and beard and feathered legs.

Belgian Bearded d'Anvers have clean legs, without the feathers, but have beards, as do the d'Uccle. Booted and d'Anvers bantams were crossed to create the d'Uccle.

Their feathery feet and legs include vulture hocks, stiff feathers growing out of the lower thighs, pointing back and down. Among clean-legged breeds, vulture hocks are unthinkable and disqualify every other breed (except Sultans) from showing, but they are a requirement in these two feather-legged breeds.

All three have feathers that are harder than breeds such as the Cochin, making them more subject to breakage. Low perches help them step up, to avoid feather damage.

They are all popular feathery bantams often seen at shows in many colors. Quail and Porcelain are unusual colors, recognized for these bantams. Mille Fleur was the original color pattern imported to the United States from Germany. These delightful little birds captivate their devotees with sparkling feathers, bright buff with black and white accents. Porcelain is a light form of Mille Fleur, cream rather than golden buff accented with blue and white.

The nuances of booted and bearded bantams take their fanciers down byways of careful breeding and meticulous care.

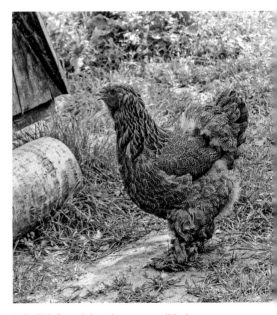

Left: This Porcelain color pattern d'Uccle rooster is as attractive as a figurine, but he's a living work of art. Although these feathery breeds are popular at poultry shows, they enjoy life in backyard flocks and lay tasty eggs. *Courtesy of the Livestock Conservancy.*
Above: *IgorSPb/Getty Images*

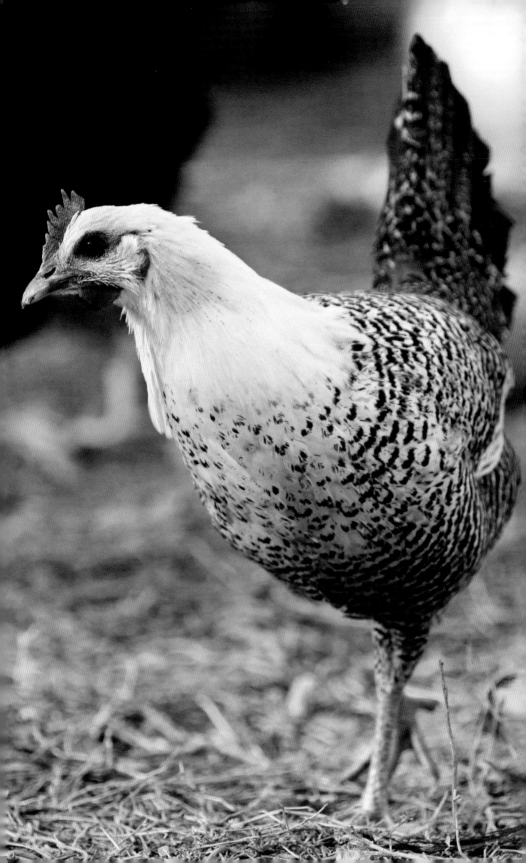

OTHER STANDARD AND NON-STANDARD BREEDS

Chickens are so varied that they defy easy classification. The APA handles this with a catch-all category, All Other Standard Breeds. The ABA has an All Other Comb Clean Leg class. The result is a mixed bag of breeds that include breeds both old and new.

Araucanas are the unusual South American chicken that lays blue eggs. That eye-catcher led to the development of the Ameraucana, a production breed that's more robust than Araucanas.

Sultans and Naked Necks have their origins in Turkey and Eastern Europe. Their unusual characteristics make them stand out visually. Naked Necks' immune system makes them resistant to many diseases. Fayoumis are the Egyptian native chicken. Rapanui fowl are native to Easter Island, off South America's coast.

Japanese breeders have developed their birds to high levels, with tails that follow them, ten feet and longer. Long crowing chickens are another refinement of chickens' many talents. Roosters may crow as long as twenty-five seconds, and the hens may crow, as well.

Norse adventurers sailed the seas hundreds of years ago, to explore and conquer. They reached lands far from their Scandinavian base, in Britain, Iceland, even North America. Of course, they brought along their chickens, and traders from other lands brought theirs to Norway and Sweden. Those chickens have come down through the centuries as unique products of history and cultural mixing.

Seramas arrived in the United States from Malaysia in 2001 and enjoyed such popularity that they were accepted into the ABA Standard only ten years later. Seramas are a small bird on a fast track.

This Fayoumi hen resembles hens that laid eggs for pharaohs in ancient Egypt. Today, her sisters in Egypt scratch out their own living. She lives a good life in a backyard flock. *Dare 2 Dream Farms*

ARAUCANA AND EASTER EGGER

Araucanas have an immediately noticeable trait: no tail! Instead, their backs slope downward. Their spine is shorter than that of other chickens, missing the last two vertebrae. That eliminates the preening (uropygial) gland as well, a disadvantage.

Their sweet faces are framed with upturned feathers. The tufts, which have been described as "rings on their ears," are actually feathery stalks on the sides of the head. Araucanas are small, at five pounds for a rooster, four pounds for a hen.

Araucanas were developed in South America in the early twentieth century, reportedly from native Collonca and Quetro chickens. The Collonca is clean-faced and rumpless, while the Quetro is tufted and tailed. Colloncas lay blue eggs, while Queteros lay pinkish-brown eggs. The patriarch of Chilean poultry, Dr. Reuben Bustos, is credited with developing Araucanas through selective breeding for the rumpless and tufted traits in the twentieth century. He called them Collonca de Aretes. The name Araucana comes from the sixteenth century Spanish name for the local Mapuche tribe, Araucanians.

They came as a surprise to North Americans in April 1927, when National Geographic published a painting of them in an issue devoted to chickens. A breeder brought the first trio to North America in 1930. Those birds were bred with others to create the birds that achieved APA recognition in 1976 and are recognized in five color varieties—Black, Black-Breasted Red, Golden Duckwing, Silver Duckwing, and White—in both large fowl and bantam. The ABA also recognizes Blue, Buff, and Silver Araucanas but not the Golden Duckwing and Silver Duckwing the APA recognizes.

Their blue eggs are irresistible, but Araucanas present difficult breeding problems. The tuft gene and the rumpless gene, if inherited from both parents, kill the chick before it hatches. Even chicks that hatch can be frail and may not survive.

The blue egg gene is dominant, so it can be bred into other breeds. Unusual color eggs are popular, and backyard fanciers enjoy keeping Easter Egger chickens that lay various colors. Those chickens do not fit any Standard definition for exhibition. They are fun and make good backyard birds, but don't qualify for chicken shows.

Show quality Araucanas are few, because both tufts and rumplessness are required, but are not reliably inherited. Chicks may hatch with single instead of double tufts, or no tufts at all. They may have tails, or small tails, or no tail. Getting both traits in one bird is the exception rather than the rule.

Easter Eggers means chickens that lay blue, green, or other pastel-color eggs. They aren't a breed, but those colorful eggs make them popular backyard chickens.
Asillem/Shutterstock

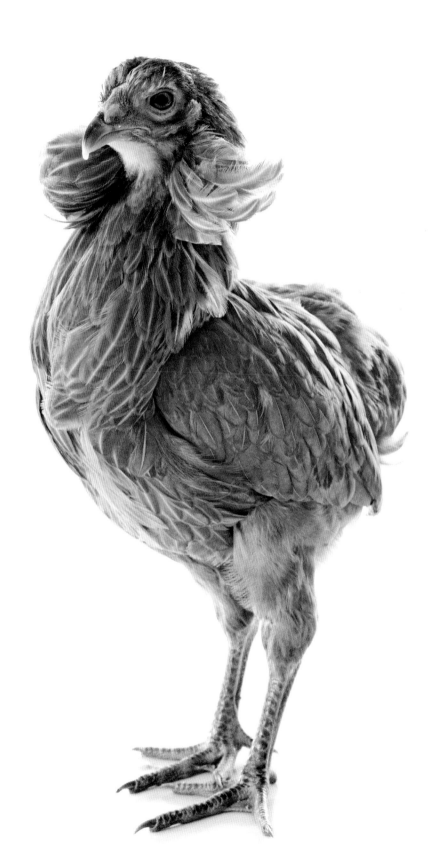

AMERAUCANA

Breeders valued Araucanas even if they had muffs and beards instead of tufts, or tails, and embarked on breeding them into a separate breed, American Araucanas, which eventually became Ameraucanas (recognized in 1984).

Ameraucanas kept the Araucana pea comb but do not have those tufts. They do have feathery faces with muffs and beards. They have full spines, tails, and preening glands.

It's considered a meat breed as well as an egg breed, although neither has the large frame of Asiatic or English meat breeds. Ameraucanas are larger than Araucanas—six and a half pounds for roosters, five and a half for hens.

Ameraucanas are recognized in eight colors by the ABA and APA, both large fowl and bantams.

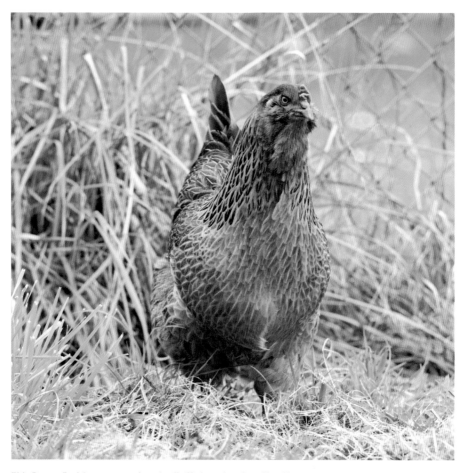

This Brown Red Ameraucana has the fluffy beard and muffs of her breed, topped by a compact pea comb. Her distinction is the blue eggs she lays. *Anna Hoychuk/Shutterstock*

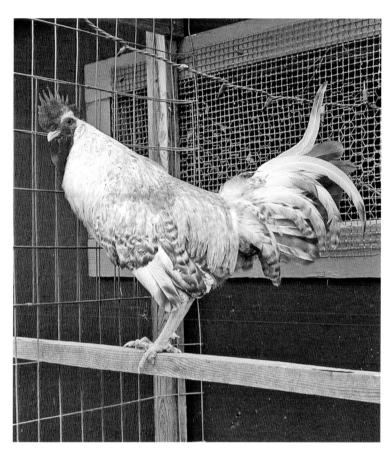

This Norwegian Jærhøn rooster has a sharp eye. That's part of his heritage as a naturally developed landrace. Jærhøn plumage isn't standardized, so a flock may have birds with varied plumage. *Barry Koffler*

JÆRHØN

Jærhøns are not much bigger than bantams. Some are light yellow and some dark brown, but the barring on their feathers isn't like the distinct barring of Standard breeds such as Plymouth Rocks. It's more like barring mixed with spots. All of them have bright yellow legs.

They are Norway's indigenous chicken, the landrace that developed from chickens that were brought to Norway. Breeders who didn't want to lose this native Norwegian chicken bred them for consistent feather color patterns in the 1920s. They are autosexing, which means that male and female chicks appear different from the day they hatch, a convenience for those who want to raise only laying hens. Jærhøns aren't recognized by the APA or the ABA.

They lay large white eggs and are considered an egg breed. While not many people keep them, they could make an attractive backyard chicken, especially for families of Norwegian ancestry. They are small and active and fly well.

ICELANDIC

No two chickens in this flock are alike. Some have single combs, some rose combs, some double combs. Some are crested, others not. Their feathering is different on every bird: different colors, mottled, barred, penciled, all kinds of markings. The roosters are much bigger than the hens, and have long spurs and long flowing tails. They are Icelandic chickens, the chickens of the Vikings.

As Vikings sailed the world in the eighth through the eleventh centuries, their chickens sailed with them. That challenging life meant that only the strongest, most adaptable, and hardiest chickens survived.

The chickens that stayed with settlers in Iceland foraged on the landscape and in the barnyard. Their descendants acquired the traits they needed to thrive in the harsh climate. The result is a landrace of chickens that are all different but all useful and valued.

Although Iceland restricts most livestock imports, White and Brown Leghorns were allowed into the country in the 1930s. They became the popular egg breed, displacing the native Icelandics. Some also bred into native flocks. Today's Icelandics have some of that Leghorn influence.

Icelandic chickens, Islenska landnámshænan, are protected in Iceland as a cultural resource. In 1974, the Agricultural Research Institute designated Icelandic chickens for special efforts to conserve the remaining native population. They are not standardized into a reliably uniform breed or recognized by either the APA or the ABA.

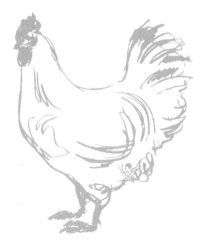

This Icelandic rooster may look very different from another Icelandic rooster and all the hens in the flock. Icelandic chickens are a landrace, not standardized as recognized chickens breeds are. They are a protected in Iceland as a cultural resource. *Courtesy of the Livestock Conservancy*

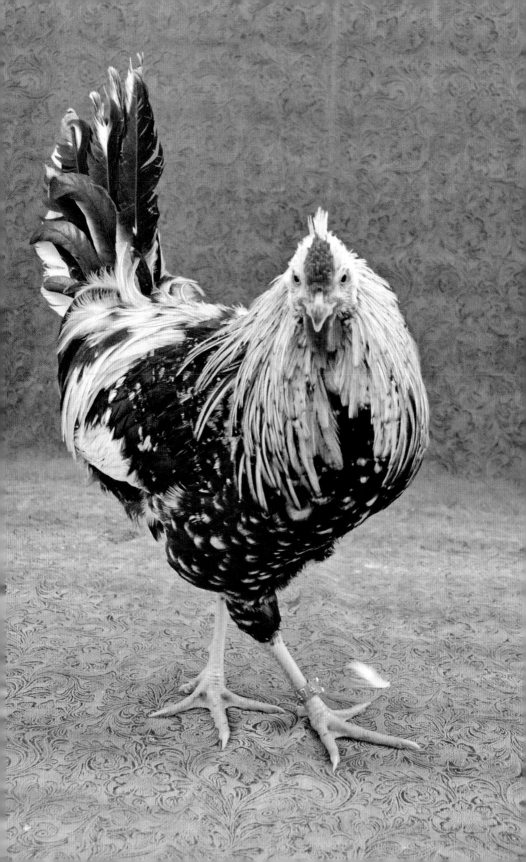

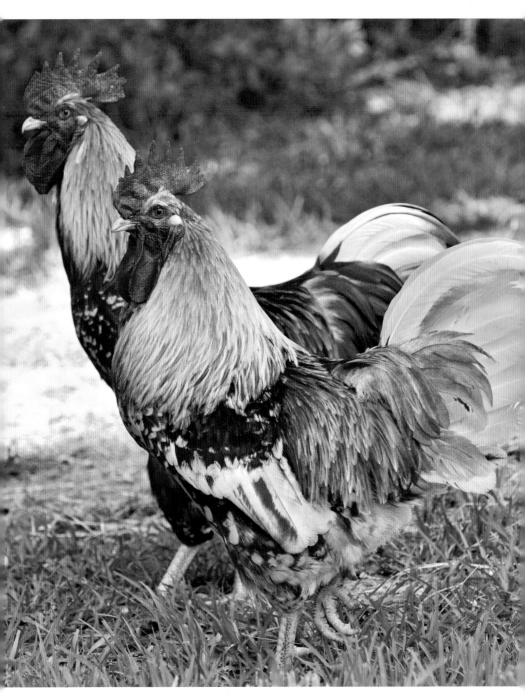

These Swedish Flower Hen roosters illustrate the wide variety of feather colors that are typical of this landrace. *Courtesy Greenfire Farms*

SWEDISH FLOWER HEN

These chickens are all colors, but every one of them has lots of white spots. White birds, and some of the gray ones, have dark spots.

Swedish Flower Hens are the traditional chickens of Sweden, Skånsk Blommehöna in Swedish, the landrace that grew in farmyards without much interference from their keepers. They have a long history, changing over the centuries as different chickens arrived in Sweden with traders and warriors.

By the late twentieth century, keepers lost interest in them and flocks gradually disappeared. Three flocks were identified, in three separate Swedish villages. Their owners dedicated themselves to saving Swedish Flower Hens from extinction. The breed organization, Svenska Lanthönsklubben, has established gene bank status for them. Organizations and farmers that keep Swedish rare breeds can get support through the Swedish rural development program.

The modern result is a chicken that is a good forager but tolerates confinement. They are good meat chickens and lay medium to large tinted eggs. Swedish Flower Hens are mild-mannered and easily tamed by handling. Although they come from a cold climate, they tolerate hot weather as well.

In the United States, a small flock of fifteen birds was imported in 2010. Their eggs and offspring have been shared with other enthusiasts. At least one breeder is working to develop an American variant. They are rare, putting prices high, but their qualities make them good backyard chickens.

Because they are not an APA Standard breed, they come in many colors and may have small crests or be clean-headed. Color patterns are vivid, described as Snow Leopard or Snowflakes on a Field.

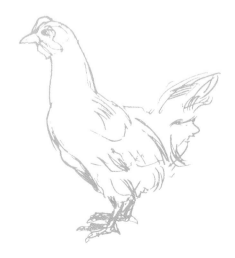

NAKED NECK

Naked Neck chickens look as if they were crossed with turkeys. Their long, skinny necks stick up, topped with a big red comb and bright red wattles hanging down.

They are sometimes called Turkens, but they aren't related to turkeys and don't have geographic relation to the country of Turkey. As unusual as they look, nakedness isn't a new trait. The naked neck gene occurs in chicken flocks around the world. The same gene also causes them to have fewer feathers all over, half the feathers of other chickens.

Fewer feathers means it's easier for them to stay cool, but they also tolerate cold weather well. They rarely get sick, apparently immune to most diseases. They lay well and make good meat birds.

Naked Necks can be any color, but only four are recognized for APA shows: Red, White, Black, and Buff. The ABA also recognizes Blue and Cuckoo. Creators of this interesting variation plan to get them to breed status and eventually recognized by the poultry organizations.

The naked gene is dominant, so it's easy to see its effects when bred into flocks of other breeds. One popular cross is the Naked Neck/Silkie, which results in a cross called Showgirls that have the bare neck topped with the Silkies' topknot of hair-like feathers. Instead of the bright red skin of Naked Necks, Showgirls retain the blue-black skin of Silkies.

Poultry scientists have used the naked gene to breed entirely featherless chickens. They look pathetic. The scientists announced their achievement with pride, but the public greeted the birds with horror. If they're being raised anywhere, their keepers are keeping them a secret.

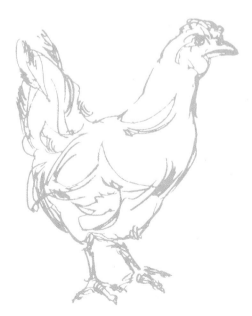

No, this Black Naked Neck is not the offspring of a chicken and a turkey! Sparse feathering is common in some breeds, and Naked Necks have only about half the feathers of other chickens.
Nataly Karol/Shutterstock

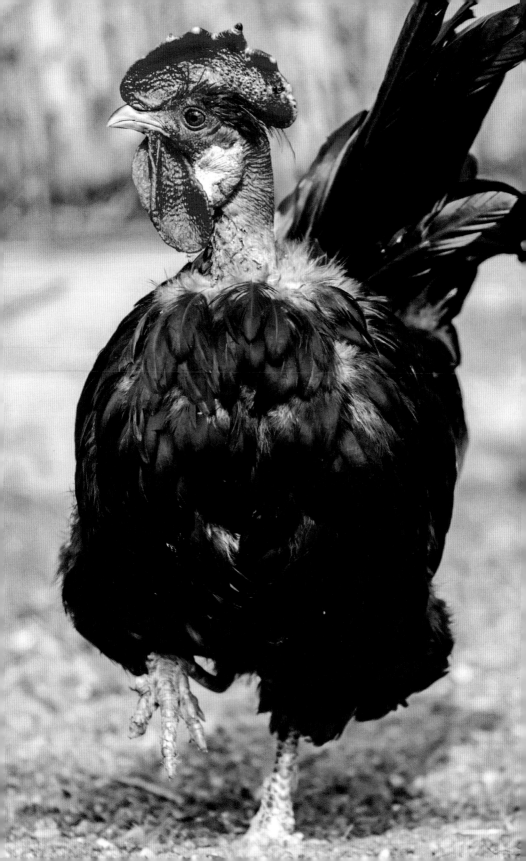

LONG CROWERS

You'll hear this chicken before you see him. His crow goes on for ten to fifteen seconds, and perhaps even longer. Long Crowers stand tall with beautiful black plumage, topped with bright red comb and wattles.

Chickens with special or unusual crows have always had special appeal. The Ayam Bekisir is a Junglefowl cross with a musical crow that Southeast Asian boatmen rely on to announce their presence to other boats in the fog. Kept in a small cage on the bow of the boat, its crowing allows sailors to keep their boats within hearing range. Turkish Denizli roosters are required to meet standards of length of crow, and their crows are judged by tone and clarity. Their performance is rated according to the position the rooster takes for his crow. The refinements are endless.

American Long Crowers come from the Japanese Tomaru breed. Tomaru are the tallest and heaviest of the long-tailed and long-crowing breeds. The most admired crow, usually ten to fifteen seconds, with the record at twenty-five seconds, is a two-tone call.

Hens have dark purple combs, and roosters' combs may be dark at the base. Roosters have long trailing sickle feathers, but they molt every year. These birds are an unusual sighting in a backyard but provide observers with a story to tell.

For the musically inclined, this Long Crower may yodel and trill for fifteen seconds or longer. Roosters' crows are the music of the barnyard, the call to bring the sun up. Long Crowers take that important job to a new level. *tunart/Getty Images*

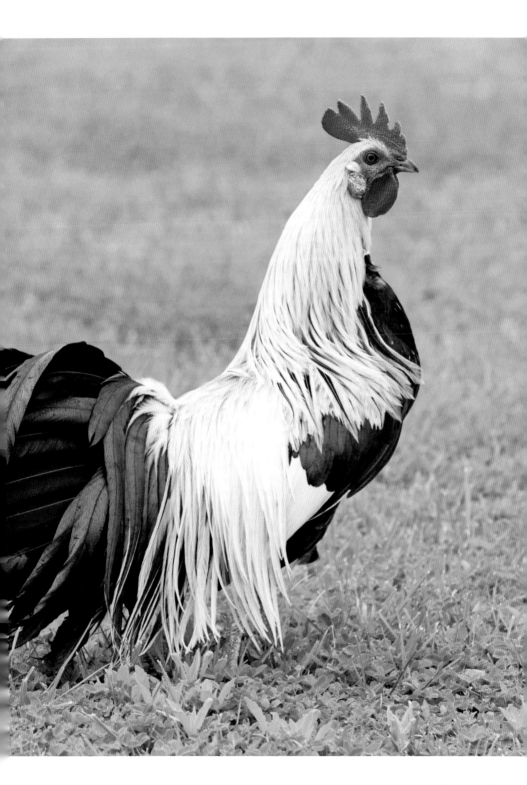

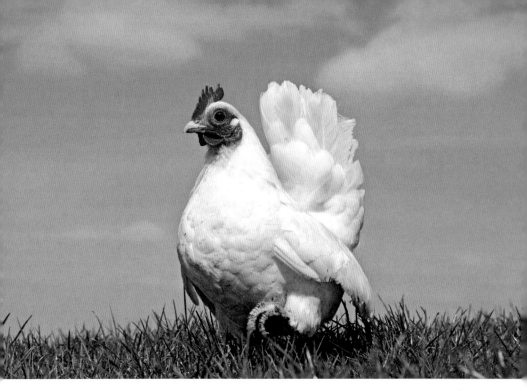

The tiny Serama is smaller than any other chicken. A Serama enthusiast's flock may include many colors, as well as white, the first color recognized. The breed is new to the United States, but its friendly nature has nestled it into bantam lovers' hearts. *Chelle129/ Shutterstock*

AMERICAN SERAMA

These tiny white chickens strut with their chests out and their tails held high. American Seramas are welcoming to visitors in their backyard and may even be found in the house, being kept as pets. Their disposition is more like a puppy's than a chicken's.

Serama fanciers raise them in a wide variety of colors. White was the first color recognized when the breed was accepted into the APA and ABA Standards in 2011. Breeders continue to work to get additional color varieties recognized. Black and Exchequer varieties are poised for recognition in 2016, followed by Wheaten in 2018.

Three types of Seramas are raised, but only the American Serama is recognized. Traditional Seramas are much like American Seramas, but breeders select birds for temperament and conformation above color of plumage, skin, eye, or earlobe. Their top weight limit is a few ounces larger than the American Serama. Ayam (Malaysian) types have higher chests and their wings are more forward than American and Traditional.

American Serama roosters weigh only sixteen ounces, hens only fourteen.

FAYOUMI

These small chickens, with silver-white heads on black-and-white barred bodies, are Egyptian Fayoumis.

They are wary of people, almost a feral chicken. They are the landrace chickens of Cairo. Fayoumis show the influence of the many traders and invaders that brought their chickens to Egypt over the centuries.

In the earliest days, Hebrews domesticated chickens into egg layers from the game chickens that arrived from India. The Egyptians welcomed this addition to the varied poultry they already kept: geese, quail, ducks, and guineafowl, about fifteen centuries BCE. Later diplomats brought Sri Lankan Junglefowl as tribute to the king. Their wild nature allowed them to catch flies in mid-air and nest in palm trees. Without the protection of poultry keepers, the survivors relied on sharp senses to warn them of predators. Brightly colored chickens that stood out against the background of bright white sand and burned gray shore and hillock were vulnerable, so Fayoumis' white heads and barred bodies suited their desert life perfectly.

Fayoumis of today live wild in many areas of Egypt. Other variants have developed in isolated settings. The danger to them now is that their landrace genes may be lost by interbreeding with modern domestic birds.

The University of Iowa maintains a flock of Fayoumis, for research on their possible natural resistance to diseases such as avian influenza, West Nile virus, malaria, and coryza.

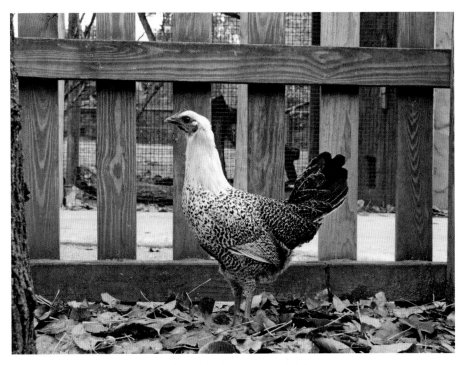

The Egyptian Fayoumi is the descendant of chickens that roamed the royal courtyards of the pharaohs. They retain some wildness in their home country but can be attractive additions to a backyard flock. *Courtesy of the Livestock Conservancy*

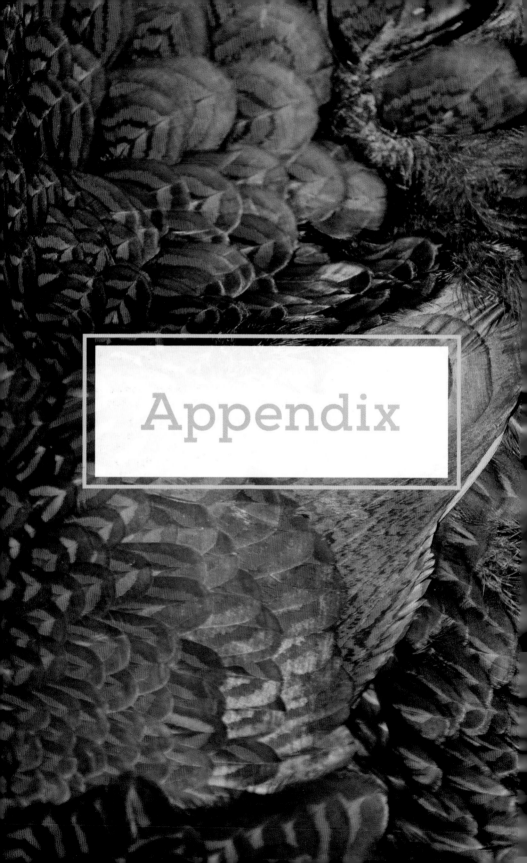

Appendix

Glossary

Color Patterns

The Standard of Perfection specifies details of feather color. The following are general definitions. To determine the exact meaning, consult the Standard.

Barred: Bars of contrasting colors on individual feathers

Laced: A border of contrasting color around the edge on individual feathers

Mottled: Some feathers tipped with white

Penciled: Concentric contrasting lines on individual feathers

Spangled: Either black or white V with a rounded end at the tip of every feather

Striped: A line of contrasting color on saddle and hackle feathers

Stippled: Contrasting dots of color

Color patterns are strictly defined in the Standard. Judges take years to master the nuances. These brief descriptions are general. Roosters and hens typically differ in intensity of colors, but some patterns are entirely different from each other.

Birchen: White head and back, with black-striped white feathers on neck and wings, becoming all black on the breast, body, and tail

Black: Pure black with greenish shine

Black Breasted Red: Traditional barnyard chicken colors, with a red golden head and neck over black breast, wings, and tail

Black-Tailed Buff: Buff head and body leading to a black tail

Blue, Self Blue: The Blue color pattern is actually laced with dark blue or black. Self Blue means solid even blue all over. Blue can replace black in many other color patterns, such as blue lacing, blue red, blue wheaten, blue quail, etc.

Brassy Back: Shades of brass on head, neck, back, and saddle with blue laced breast, body, and wings with some blue feathers, leading to a blue tail

Buff: Golden buff all over

Columbian: Mostly white with black and white cape and a black tail

Dark: Greenish black with some dark red spots on back and saddle feathers

Dark Brown: Rooster is red in head, hackle, back, and saddle, with black breast, body, and tail. Wings are red and black. Hen is reddish bay with black stippling leading to a black tail topped by two feathers stippled with red brown. Her wings are black with red brown stippling.

Exchequer: Black and white evenly distributed over the whole bird

Golden: Rooster has a creamy white head and neck, with black stripes on the neck and saddle feathers. A golden back leads to black breast, body, and tail. Black wings with some white accents. Hen's head, hackle, back, and body are various shades of gray and stippling in some sections over a salmon breast. Her tail is mainly black, with two gray stippled feathers on top. Her wings are mostly stippled gray with brown primaries.

Golden Duckwing: Rooster has a creamy white head and neck over a light golden back and black breast, body, and wings. Wings have black shoulders and fronts, with golden bows, coverts barred with bluish black, primaries edged with white, and secondaries barred with creamy white. Hen has a gray head and body, with salmon on the front of her neck and gray with brownish black stripes on the back. Her back is gray feathers stippled with lighter gray, her breast is salmon, and her wings have some gray feathers stippled with lighter gray and some dark brown.

Golden Laced and Silver Laced: Golden or white feathers with black edging or stripes all over leading to a black tail

Gray: Silvery white with some black striped feathers over a black breast, body, and tail, with black and white wings

Lemon Blue: Lemon on head, back, and saddle, with dark blue feathers laced with lemon

Light: White head, back, saddle, and breast, with black hackles edged with silvery white and a black tail

Light Brown: Lots of reddish orange with some black edges on head, neck, and back, leading to a black breast, body, and tail

Mille Fleur: Each bright orange red feather has a black stripe and a white spangle tip

Partridge: Red head and wings, with black feathers shimmering with red edges on back, saddle, and tail coverts, and black breast, body, and tail

Porcelain: Each feather beige tipped with white spangle and a blue bar

Quail: Rooster is mostly black with golden bay highlights. His breast and body are covered in brownish yellow feathers laced with darker yellow, and his tail is black. The hen is mostly chocolate black laced with bay. Her breast and body are brownish yellow laced with lighter yellow. Her wings are black.

Red Pyle: Bright orange head, neck, and back, over a white breast, body, and tail

Red Shoulder: Rooster is white, with a reddish breast and blood red wing bows and coverts. Hen is white with salmon breast and back. Her wing bows and coverts are salmon tipped with white spangles.

Salmon: Rooster has a light straw yellow head, neck, and saddle over a brown red back, and black breast, body, and tail, with brown red wing feathers laced with brass, over black, and black and white feathers. The hen is brownish salmon, salmon pink, and white.

Silver: Silvery white with some black stripes in hackle, saddle, and wings, over a black breast and body and black-and-white tail

Silver Duckwing: Rooster is white with black breast, body, wings, and tail, with some white edging on wing feathers. Hen is silvery gray with black striping on neck, stippling on her back, body, and the top two tail feathers on her black tail. She has a salmon breast.

Silver Penciled: White head over black breast, body, wings, and tail. Neck, back, and saddle feathers have white at the edges.

Speckled: Mahogany bay feathers with black stripes and white spangles. A black tail with a white tip.

Splash: Blue and white unevenly splashed on the feathers

Wheaten: Light orange to bright red on head, neck, and back, with black breast, body, and tail. Wings are black and red.

White: Pure white with a lustrous sheen

Feather Terms

Axial feather: Short wing feather between primaries and secondaries

Back: Base of the neck to the base of the tail, including cape and saddle

Beard: Fluffy feathers on the throat

Cape: Short feathers forming a cape where neck and back meet

Ear tuft: Feathers on a little tab of skin below the ear

Fluff: Downy part of a feather

Hackle: Feathers on the back and sides of the neck. Hens' have rounded edges; roosters' have pointed ones.

Muff: Feathers around the throat

Primaries: Flight feathers—the long wing feathers—concealed when the wing is folded

Saddle: Rear part of the back extending to the tail

Secondaries: Long, broad wing feathers visible when the wing is folded

Sickle: Two top feathers on the tail

Tail Covert: Curved feathers at the front and side of the tail

Tassels: Feathers growing from the back of the head behind the comb (also called topins)

Wing bow: Upper portion of the wing between the shoulder and the coverts

Wing covert: Double row of broad feathers in the middle of the wing

Feather Descriptions

Close feathered: Holding the feathers close to the body

Frizzle: Curled feathers

Hard feathers: Closely webbed and have little fluff. Typical of game breeds.

Hennies: Varieties in which the roosters resemble the hens in plumage. Ideally, the henny rooster is identical to the hen in plumage but larger in size. Henny roosters may vary from the ideal plumage–a rooster might have cock-like sickle, hackle, or saddle feathers.

Molt: The process of replacing old feathers with new. Most species change feathers once annually but some change twice. Long-tailed breeds molt only every two or three years.

Soft feathers: Loosely webbed and fluffy, typical of Asiatic breeds

Other Terms

Beetle brows: Heavy overhanging eyebrows

Capon: A castrated male. Capons do not develop the typical rooster feathering but grow large and are intended as large roasting table birds.

Carriage: The bearing, pose, or style of a breed

Condition: The state of a bird's health, reflected in its bright comb, earlobe, and face color. Clean plumage and feet. Show preparation.

Defect: A quality that makes a bird less than perfect but within the scope of competition

Disqualification: A defect so serious that the bird will not be judged

Faking: Anything that is done to mask a defect or disqualification in a bird entered in a show

Leader: The spike at the back of a rose comb

Lopped comb: A comb that falls over to one side

Sexual dimorphism: Males and females look different. Roosters are larger than hens, have bigger combs and wattles, and grow larger tails.

Trio: A male and two females of the same breed and variety

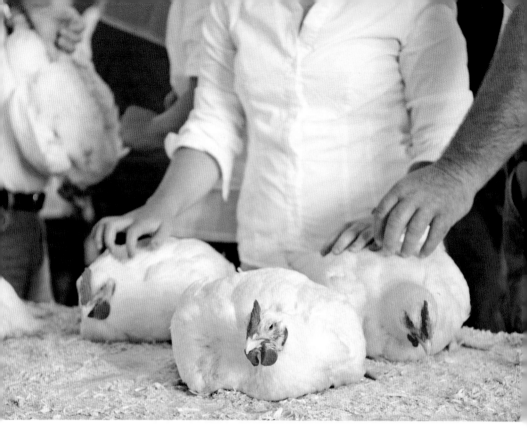

Chicken shows give proud owners a chance to show off their chickens and their expertise. 4-H and FFA hold special competitions for students. They are a great place for novices to learn about all aspects of chicken keeping. *lenda/Shutterstock*

Showing Chickens

Whether you plan to show your chickens or are attending a show to look at the chicken possibilities, learning to read the cage cards will help. They are written in a shorthand that requires some deciphering.

Chickens are judged according to the way they are classified by the American Poultry Association and the American Bantam Association. Consult the APA Standard of Perfection and the ABA Bantam Standard for all the details.

The card reads:

Class: **Variety:**
Breed: **Sex:**

The APA classes for large fowl chickens are American, Asiatic, English, Mediterranean, Continental, and the catch-all class, All Other Standard Breeds (shortened to AOSB).

Bantams have their own classes: Modern Game, Old English Game, American Game, Single Comb Clean Leg (SCCL), Rose Comb Clean Leg (RCCL), All Other Comb Clean Leg (AOCCL), and Feather Legged (FLEG). It's an alphabet soup of letters, but the logic is to keep similar birds together.

Signs indicating where the various classes are caged are often placed on top of cages or in another easily seen location. The signs will help you identify which breeds are on display.

Next is the breed. Within each class are separate breeds. Chickens are judged against others of their breed. Breeds are grouped together but may be identified only on the cage cards.

Next is the variety. Within the breed are varieties. These are usually different colors, but varieties may also be identified by different combs.

Sex seems obvious, but for chicken shows, young birds are judged separately from mature birds. Males under a year old are cockerels, females under a year old are pullets. Males over a year are cocks and females over a year are hens.

The chicken owner exhibiting the bird is identified only by a number. This helps keep judging fair and impartial.

The row of cages will be closed off while the judges are inspecting the birds. It's not necessarily solemn, but it is serious. Judges spend years studying chickens and learning the refinements of body shape, feather condition and color, comb, wattles and earlobes, and all the other points that go into judging chickens. They need to be left alone to focus on each bird.

Judges love chickens and are eager to help others learn about them. They will happily answer questions after they are finished judging.

The judge examines each bird in the variety, breed, and class, and then ranks them. Number 1, 2, and 3 rank the top three birds of that sex, variety, and breed. BV stands for Best of Variety. RV stands for Reserve of Variety, second place. BB stands for Best of Breed, meaning of all the chickens of that breed shown, all varieties, this chicken was the best. RB is Reserve of Breed, second place.

CH means champion and RCH reserve champion, second place. Champions will be awarded for each class. Up to this point, similar birds are judged against each other. The next level is judging all bantams and all large fowl, to choose champions for each group.

The champions of bantams and large fowl go to the front of the show, Champions Row. If waterfowl and turkeys are included in the show, their champions will be on Champions Row as well. From that lineup, the Grand Champion (GCH)

and the Reserve Grand Champion (RGCH) of the entire show will be selected.

Every chicken owner who goes to the trouble of preparing birds to take to a show is proud to be there. They are all proud of their birds, as you may be some day. Compliment them and ask them about their birds. Shows are an excellent way to connect with other chicken owners.

Most shows have a sale section. Most of the birds will be show quality or close to show quality. Expect to pay more than you would for less carefully bred birds. You may find some bargains.

From experience I can tell you that it is difficult to leave a show without a few new birds. I've tried limiting myself by vowing not to waver, and not bringing any empty cages with me to the show. However, chickens don't mind traveling to a new home in plain cardboard boxes.

Chicken Show Classifications for Bantams

The American Poultry Association has a Bantam division, divided into five categories for exhibition: Games, Single Comb Clean Legged Other Than Games, Rose Comb Clean Legged, All Other Combs Clean Legged, and Feather Legged. They are usually shortened to initials only at shows, resulting in an alphabet soup of letters—SCCL, RCCL, AOCCL—that looks obscure to the uninitiated. Now you know.

The American Bantam Association has its own separate standard. Although the two organizations work together cooperatively, the ABA recognizes some different breeds and more color varieties of breeds than the APA: 56 breeds and 392 varieties. The ABA divides Bantam chickens into six classes: Modern Games; Old English and American Games; Single Comb Clean Leg; Rose Comb Clean Leg; All Other Combs Clean Leg; and Feather Leg. Exhibiting bantams at shows is part of the fun of owning them.

Index

Ameraucana, 188
American Bantam Association
    Bantam Standard, 16
    breed recognition process, 17
    recent breed additions, 18
    website, 21
American breeds, 85
American Games, 69
American hybrids, 108
American Poultry Association
    breed recognition process, 17
    flock certification, 23
    recent breed additions, 18
    Standard of Perfection, 16
    website, 21
American Serama, 198
Amprolium, 53
anatomy, 33–35
ancient cultures, 14–15, 125
Ancona, 158
Andalusian, 157
antibiotics, 55–56, 59, 61
Appenzeller Spitzhauben, 146
Araucana, 15, 186
Aseel, 79
Asiatic breeds, 111
Australorp, 134
avian influenza (AI), 60

Bacitracin, 53
backyard chickens. See chicken keeping
bantams, Mediterranean breed types and,
    149
Barnevelder, 166
Belgian Bearded d'Anvers bantams, 183
Belgian Bearded d'Uccle bantams, 183
biosecurity, 59
bloodlines, 16
Booted bantams, 183
Brabanter, 146
Brahma, 112
breed clubs, websites and, 21
breed types
    American breeds, 85
    American hybrids, 108
    Asiatic breeds, 111
    Continental, 165
    crested, 139
    English breeds, 125
    Games, 65
    Mediterranean, 149
    Oriental Games, 71
    other classifications, 185
    sex-links, 109
breeding
    defining breeds, 16

heritage chickens, 17
    selective breeding, 15–16
breeds
    bloodlines, 16
    composite breeds, 16
    defining, 16
    for egg production, 26
    foundation breeds, 16
    hybrids, 16
    landraces, 16
    Livestock Conservancy ranking, 18, 21
    selecting, 19, 21
    traditional, 18–19
    varieties, 16
British Poultry Standards, 125
broilers, 29
brooding, 39–41
Buckeye, 97

Campine, 167
Catalana del Prat Leonada, 162
Chantecler, 98–99
chick starter, 53
chicken keeping
    considerations, 43
    diseases, 56, 59
    emergency preparedness, 51
    flocks, 45, 59
    heat and, 59
    illness, 60–61
    local ordinances, 44–45
    safe handling, 45
    space, 59
    water, 55, 56, 59
    yards for, 50–51
    See also coops; feed
chicken scratch, 55
coccidiosis, 53, 60
Cochin, 114
combs, 33, 61, 139
coops
    cleaning, 49
    designs and components, 46–47
    isolated spaces in, 49
    nest boxes, 48, 49
    perches, 49
    predators and, 45–46
    ventilation, 49
Cornish, 128
Crèvecoeur, 141
Cubalaya, 75

Delaware, 104
diatomaceous earth (DE), 50–51
digestive system, 36–37
diseases, 56, 59, 60–61
domestication
    of chickens, 13–15
    difficulties of, 13
Dominique, 88–89

Dorking, 126
dust-bathing, 50–51
Dutch bantams, 181

Easter Egger, 186
eggs
    of Araucanas, 15
    breeds for, 26, 30
    color of, 26
    fertilization of, 38–39
    hatching, 39–41
    of Junglefowl birds, 14
    laying process, 37–38
    nutrition and backyard, 26
    sizes, 28
    xanthophyll, 59
emergencies, 51
English breeds, 125
exhibiting chickens, 25

Faverolles, 176
Fayoumi, 199
feathers, 35–36
feed
    antibiotics and, 55–56
    chick starter, 53
    chicken diet, 53
    chicken scratch, 55
    commercial, 53
    crumble/mash, 54
    greens, 54–55
    grower, 54
    herbs, 55
    medicated, 53
    treats, 54
first-aid kits, 51
flock instinct, 45, 59
fryers, 29–30

Hamburg, 171
Hatcheries, 21
Hen Fever, 111
herbs, 55
heritage chickens, 17
Houdan, 142

Icelandic, 190
illness, 60–61
infections, 60
influenza, 60
injuries, 60
Internet, utilizing, 21–23
Iowa Blue, 105

Japanese bantam, 122–123
Jærhøn, 189
Java, 93
Jersey Giant, 101
Junglefowl birds
    domestication of, 13–15

profile, 118–119

Ko Shamo, 83
Kraienkoppe, 173

La Fleche, 175
Lakenvelder, 172
landraces, 16
Langshan, 117
Leghorn, 150
lice, 60
Livestock Conservancy, 18, 21
local ordinances, 44–45
Long Crowers, 196

Malays, 72
Manure, 25, 30–31
Marans, 179
mating process, 38–39
meat
    breeds for, 30
    categorization by age, 29–30
    cooking methods, 26, 28
    egg breeds and, 30
    flavor and, 28–29
medicinal uses, 14
Minorca, 153
mites, 60, 61
Modern Games, 68

Naked Neck, 194
New Hampshire, 102
Normandy fowl, 142

Old English Games, 67
Onigadori, 76–77
Oriental Games, 71
Orloffs, 81
Orpington, 130–131

Penedesenca, 163
Phoenix chickens, 76–77
Plymouth Rock, 87
Polish, 140
predators, 45–46
prognostication, 14
Pyncheon bantam, 106

Red Junglefowl
    colors of, 14
    domestication of, 13–15
    eggs of, 14
    Junglefowl profile, 118–119
    original size of, 13
Redcap, 135
Rhode Island Red/White, 94
roasters, 30
rodents, 59
Rosecomb bantam, 136
Russian Orloff, 81

salmonella, 60
scaly leg mites, 61
Sebright bantam, 137
sex-links, 109
Shamo, 82
Sicilian Buttercup, 161
Silkie, 120
Skånsk Blommehöna, 193
social media, 22–23
strains, 16
succession plans, 51
Sulmtaler, 145
Sultan, 147
Sumatra, 73
Sussex, 133
Swedish Flower Hen, 193

traditional breeds
  about, 18–19
  vs. hybrid industrial chickens, 22
treats, 54

varieties, 16
veterinarians, 61
Vorwerk bantam, 107

waste disposal, 25
water, 55, 56, 59
Welsummer, 169
White-Faced Black Spanish, 154
Wyandotte, 90–91

Yokohama, 78

About the Author

Christine Heinrichs is a member of the American Poultry Association, the American Bantam Association, and the Livestock Conservancy. She grew up in suburban New Jersey but moved to rural California in the 1980s. Her daughter's plea for baby chicks started her on her poultry journey.

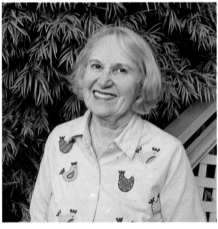

She holds a degree in journalism from the University of Oregon and is a member of the Society of Professional Journalists, the Society of Environmental Journalists, Northern California Science Writers Association, and Ten Spurs, the honorary society of the Mayborn Literary Nonfiction Conference. She is the author of *How to Raise Chickens* and *How to Raise Poultry*. Her magazine articles have been published in a wide range of magazines, from *Backyard Poultry* to *Audubon*.

She lives with her husband, cat, and chickens in California.